Dr. K. E. SHARIAN
1974

INTRODUCTION TO ACUPUNCTURE ANESTHESIA

WILLIAM C. LOWE, M.D., M.Sc. (Med.)

Assistant Professor of Medicine
College of Medicine and Dentistry of New Jersey
New Jersey Medical School

MEDICAL EXAMINATION PUBLISHING COMPANY, INC.
65-36 Fresh Meadow Lane
Flushing, N.Y. 11365

Copyright © 1973 by the Medical Examination Publishing Co., Inc.

Copyright © 1973 by the Medical Examination Publishing Co., Inc.

All rights reserved. No part of this publication may be reproduced in any form or by any means, electronic or mechanical, including photocopy, without permission in writing from the publisher.

Library of Congress
Catalog Card Number
76-115121

ISBN 0-87488-753-4

JUNE, 1973

PRINTED IN THE UNITED STATES OF AMERICA

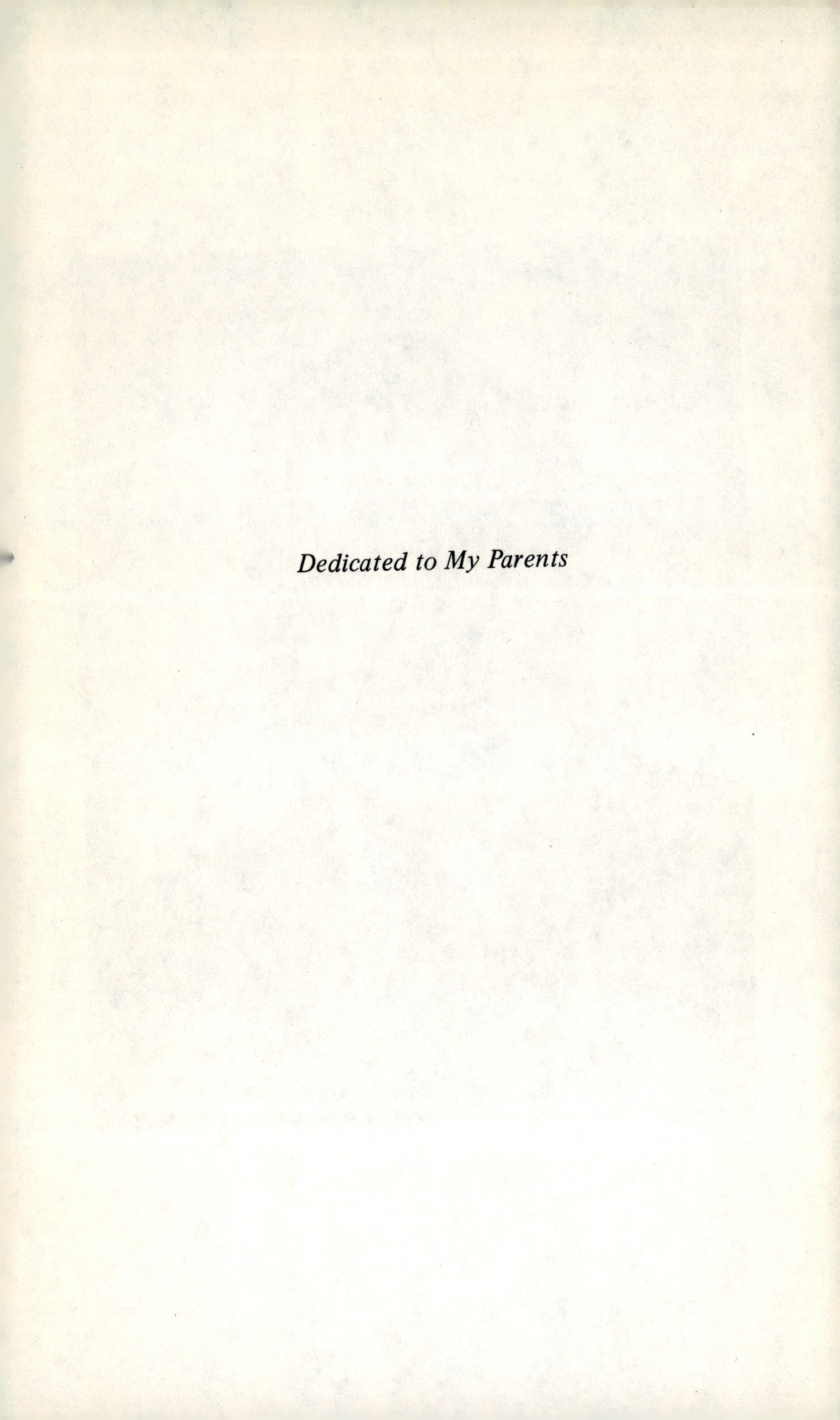

Dedicated to My Parents

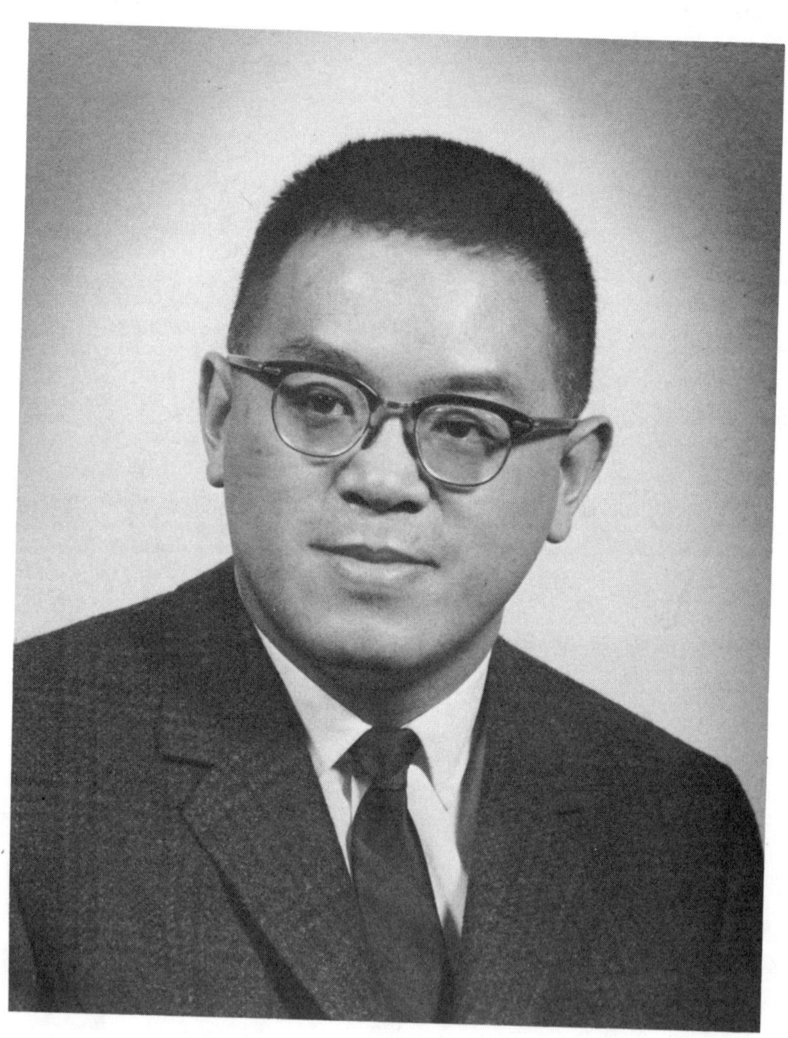

ABOUT THE AUTHOR

Dr. Lowe graduated from the National Medical College of Shanghai, China, and interned at the Queen Mary Hospital, Hong Kong and Jersey City Medical Center. He received his postgraduate medical education at the University of Pennsylvania and Temple University Schools of Medicine in Philadelphia. He is at present Assistant Professor of Medicine at the College of Medicine and Dentistry of New Jersey – New Jersey Medical School, and Acting Chief, Oncology Section at the Veterans Administration Hospital, East Orange, New Jersey. He has had numerous articles published in leading professional journals and is the author of the book "Neoplasms of the Gastrointestinal Tract", published by the Medical Examination Publishing Company, Inc., Flushing, N.Y.

PREFACE

This book represents an effort of collecting and editing recent literature on acupuncture anesthesia published throughout the world, especially from China. A large amount of material was reviewed and only articles with possible scientific merit were included. Since most of the acupuncture articles from China were not published in the professional journals, the information may appear to be somewhat anecdotal according to the Western standards. However, these abundant factual observations are valuable assets which may lay the groundwork for future experimentation and improvement of acupuncture in this country.

During my preparation of the book, it was comforting to note that the neurosurgeons and neurologists were in general much less skeptical and much more receptive to the concepts of acupuncture than the local physicians and surgeons.

In chapter XII, the concepts of electroanalgesia were presented. This is a technique of stimulating the dorsal column of the spinal cord or the peripheral nerve by a pulsating electric current and is evidently effective in treating certain chronic pain syndromes. The only criticism is that this technique requires prolonged contact of the electrode with the nervous structure, which may result in permanent damage. Although damage to the nervous system has been emphatically denied by neurosurgeons in human and animal experiments, the fear of such damage nevertheless persists. The concepts of electroanalgesia, however, seem to be perfect for acupuncture, which only requires a temporary effect in relieving pain from the operation.

The effect of acupuncture appears without doubt, in my opinion, to be mediated through the peripheral and the central nervous systems. I sincerely hope that the information provided in this book may help to open new fields of research in the treatment of such diseases as hypertension, neuralgias, mental disorders, deaf-mutism, among others.

I wish to thank the many faculty members of our institution for their enthusiastic support, without which the book could never have been completed. First, I wish to express my gratitude to Miss Carole A. Hall, our librarian, for her ability and effort to obtain every acupuncture article quoted in the Index Medicus, and to Mrs. Virginia Campan for her painstaking correction of my manuscript. Secondly, I am grateful to Dr. Francis F. Chinard and Dr. Norman H. Ertel of the Department of Medicine; Dr. Stuart D. Cook and Dr. Raymond A. Troiano of the Department of Neurology; Dr. Allan Siegel of the Department of Anatomy and Dr. Henry M. Edinger of the Department of Physiology for their comments, criticisms, and assistance. I also wish to thank Mr. Stanley Schwartz, the medical artist, for producing all necessary illustrations, and to our efficient secretaries, Mrs. Kathleen A. Cimino and Miss Patricia A. Leppin for their typing and retyping of the manuscript. Lastly, I am most grateful to Mr. David C. Dimendberg of the Medical Examination Publishing Company for his understanding, suggestion, and counselling in the publication of this book.

Since this book summarizes data which have not been gathered by standard controlled methods used in Western countries, it is important to stress that the conclusions cited do not reflect the views of the College of Medicine and Dentistry of New Jersey – New Jersey Medical School.

WILLIAM C. LOWE, M.D.
South Orange, N.J.

INTRODUCTION TO ACUPUNCTURE ANESTHESIA

TABLE OF CONTENTS

CHAPTER

CHAPTER I

INTRODUCTION

Acupuncture is the science of inserting sharp needles into certain points of the body and achieving the desired therapeutic result either by mechanical stimulation with manual turning and twirling of the needle, or by electrical stimulation with the application of a direct pulsating current.

No one knows exactly when acupuncture began in China. In the Yellow Emperor's Classic of Internal Medicine,[1] published some 2400 years ago, there were already detailed descriptions of the needles used in acupuncture and of the various points in the body where it could be used most effectively. Theories were also provided to explain the mechanisms by which acupuncture worked on the body. It seemed that inflicting injuries or wounds by striking certain parts of the body with sharpened stones had a "curative" effect on a specific illness from which the individual had suffered for a long time.[2–7] For example, a wound on a specific part of the foot would relieve a headache or toothache; a wound below the knee joint would cure a stomachache. All these observations were noted collectively and confirmed over many centuries. As time went on, it was noted, however, that neither the size nor the depth of the wound was important. What was important was the exact location on the skin where the wound should be made. It was quite effective when the wound was only one-tenth of an inch in diameter.[8]

In the early days, sharpened fish bones or bamboo shafts were used to perform acupuncture. When metal was discovered, needles sharpened to a fine point were used.[9] The needles were first made of gold or silver, but because of their cost, only wealthy people could afford to use them.

In the course of many centuries, hundreds of acupuncture points were recorded, each one named after its discoverer.[3] Books were written describing the exact location of these points and the various diseases, from back pains to toothaches, that could be cured by their stimulation. Special departments of acupuncture were established in early Chinese schools of medicine. In the beginning of the nineteenth century, however, the practice of acupuncture fell into dispute among modern Western-trained doctors. Practitioners of Chinese folk medicine kept acupuncture alive among the general population, although it was obviously forbidden in the modern, more sophisticated hospitals.[10-13]

The total number of acupuncture points on the body varied, depending upon the reviewer. For example, 365 points were recorded in the Yellow Emperor's Classic of Internal Medicine,[1] and only 160 points were given in literature published in the Han dynasty.[10-13] The French workers, probably as a result of their more exhaustive reviews, reported approximately 800 points of acupuncture.[3] The total number of reported points is perhaps not as important as the knowledge of the exact location of the more senstive, and therefore, more effective points.

As in any branch of science, when certain facts are known, theories are proposed to explain the phenomenon. According to the Chinese tradition, the acupuncture points are divided into twelve main groups, all the points in one group being united by a line called the meridian. The meridian, in turn, connects with certain organs of the body so that "the interior of the body has a relationship with the external environment." Then there are theories of the flow of energy, the equilibrium of two vital principles such as Yin and Yang, and the five elements of nature exemplified in metal, wood, water, fire, and earth. As long as certain proportions of the various parts of the body remain normal, the body will be healthy; any disturbance in the balance results in disease.

It must be noted that these theories were proposed many thousands of years ago when scientific information was lacking. Their accurancy and reliability are open to question.[14-21] To study them as matter of historic interest is logical, but to use them as the sole basis in favor of acupuncture appears to be unwarranted.

CHAPTER II

THE NEEDLES

It is of no great importance what material is used in making acupuncture needles. The main objective is to stimulate the chosen points.[2] The needles have undergone refinement through the centuries from sharpened stone, then bamboo or fishbone, to gold and silver. The most serviceable metal, however, is stainless steel. In fact, the most frequently used needles in China and European countries today are made of stainless steel.[2 2–2 5]

There are many types of needles. (Figs. 1 and 2) A triangular-shaped needle is used for releasing blood; a round needle is used for massage; a skin needle is mainly employed for children. The skin needle is a small mallet with six or seven small needles clustered in an area of approximately one square centimeter. The procedure is to hold the handle of the needle and tap the points on the skin rhythmically for three to five times. The heaviness of the stroke depends upon the sensitivity of the skin in that area. The skin needle is usually applied on the back and flank regions at first, then the four extremities, and on the painful areas last.

The most commonly used needles for insertion, the haochen, consist of three parts: a handle with fine wire wound thickly around it, a neck, and the needle itself with its sharp point. There are different lengths of needles: ½″, 1″, 3″, 4″, 5″, 6″, and 8″; and four sizes: Nos. 26, 28, 30, and 32. The most popular needles are 1½″ in length and Nos. 28 and 30.

The needles must meet certain requirements of quality and cost. They must be very fine and flexible. Under no

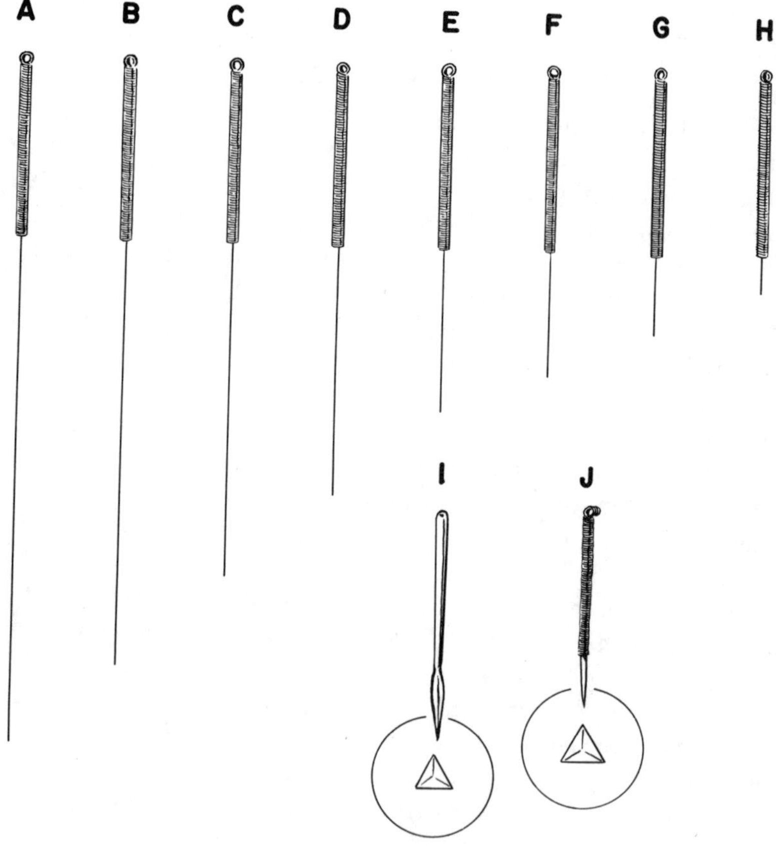

Fig. 1 Acupuncture needles. Hao-chen A, B, C, D, E, F, G, H are of lengths 6″, 5″, 4′, 3″, 2″, 1½″, 1″, and ½″ respectively. I and J are triangular-shaped needles with magnified views of their tips.

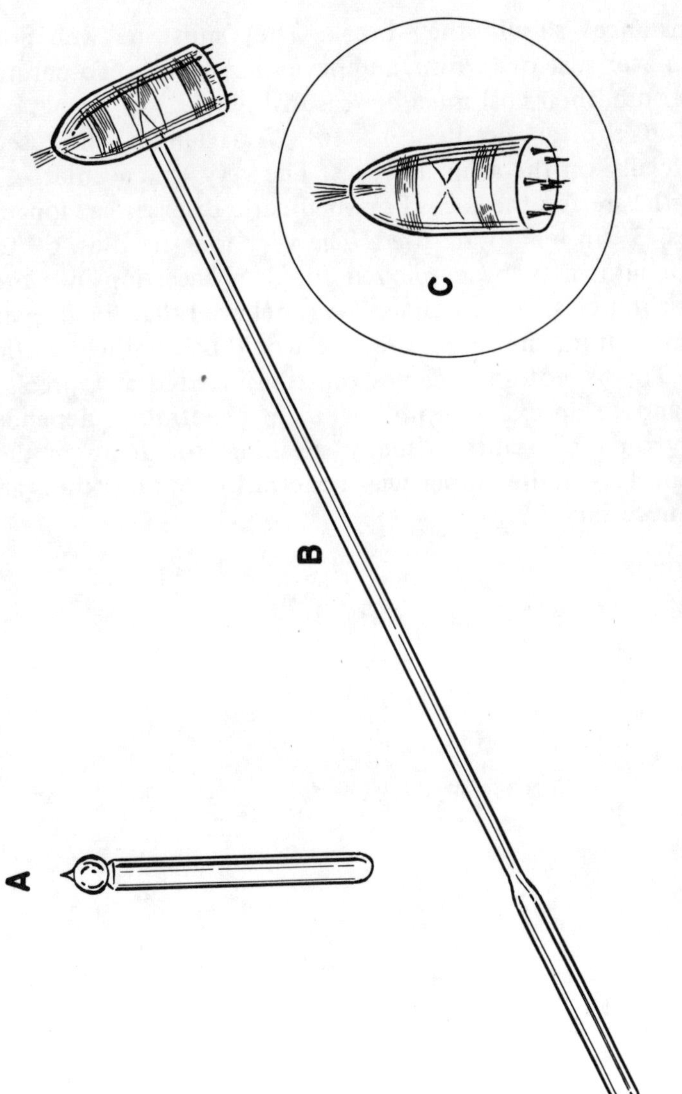

Fig. 2 A. Round needle for massage. B. Plastic skin needle for children. C. Mallet with seven small needles clustered in one end.

circumstances should they break. They must be well polished, never rust or tarnish, and have sharp points. To permit popular use, their cost must be reasonably low.

The shorter needles, 1″ to 2″ in length, are used superficially on the arms and legs. The very fine needles, ½″ in length, are for the face. For rheumatic disease, the longer needles, 3″ in length are used. The very long needles, 6″ to 8″ in length, may be employed for deep insertion into the buttock muscles. At one time, it was believed that the deeper the penetration, the more effective would be the therapeutic result. This is not so. Needles must be inserted at a precise point and to an exact depth. Depth of penetration depends entirely on the locality. Usually speaking, for areas on the arms and legs, rather superficial penetration of the skin is all that is necessary.[25]

CHAPTER III

TECHNIQUES OF ACUPUNCTURE

A. Preliminary Practice

As the first consideration is to minimize pain from insertion of the needle, the acupuncturist must see that the needle is straight, not rusted, and its point sharp. If this is not the case, a new needle should be used. Preliminary practice to improve the operator's skill in acupuncture is necessary so that the procedure will be comfortable for the patient. Developing strength in inserting the needle and skill in twirling it are prerequisites of good acupuncture techniques.[22–25]

1. To develop strength in inserting the needle (Fig. 3): Fold up ten or twelve sheets of paper toweling, and fasten the pile of paper with paper tapes. Hold the pile of paper in the left hand. Insert the needle into the paper with a decisive and quick stroke. Such a stroke used on a patient would be less painful than a hesitant and slow maneuver. Practice first with a half-inch needle. Then, when your technique improves, practice with 1″, 2″, or 3″ needles. Hold the needles with the thumb, index, and middle fingers of the right hand. Use a slight twirling movement to facilitate quick penetration of the paper pile. Practice repeatedly until the procedure becomes natural and effortless.

2. To develop skill in twirling the needle (Fig. 4): The best practice is to make a cotton ball, two or three inches in diameter. Wrap 12 or 16-ply cotton twine around the cotton ball ten times or more. Hold the ball in the left hand, and

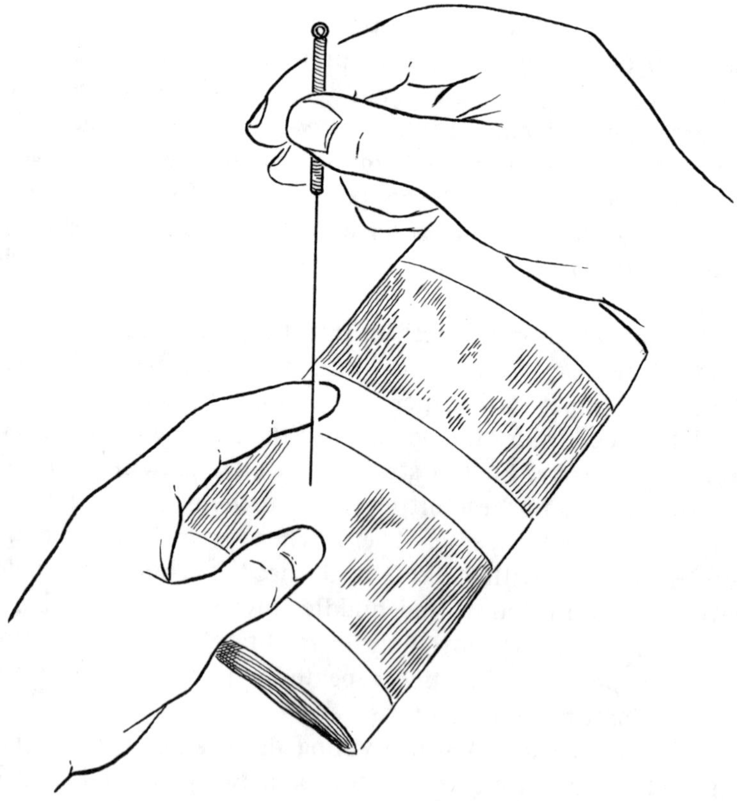

Fig. 3 Insert the needle into a pile of paper towels.

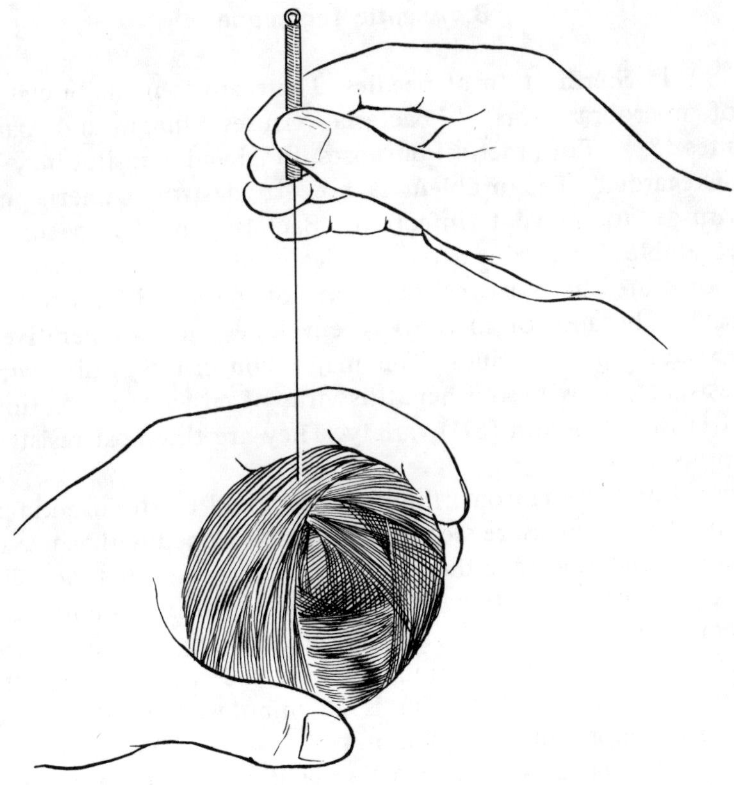

Fig. 4 Insert the needle in a ball of cotton twine.

hold the needle with the thumb, index, and middle fingers of the right hand. Practice inserting, withdrawing, and turning the needle clockwise and counterclockwise. Try combining these movements.

To gain skill, wrap the cotton ball with cotton twine more than ten times every day, and practice the above described movements diligently. As the ball gradually gets larger, skill in twirling the needle correspondingly improves. With repeated practice, the procedure becomes virtually automatic.[22]

B. Aseptic Technique

1. Sterilization of needles. There are four major classes of microorganisms – bacteria, viruses, fungi, and parasites.[26,27] For practical purposes, fungi and parasites may be disregarded. The problem is how to destroy bacteria and viruses to prevent infection. Bacteria usually occur in vegetable forms, but a few species produce spores. Bacterial spores are the most resistant form of microbe life. Tubercle bacilli, because of their waxy envelopes, are comparatively resistant to germicides. The major concern regarding viral resistance is with the hepatitis virus of either the infectious (IH) or the serum (SH) variety. They are the most resistant forms of virus.

For these reasons, the needles should be sterilized in an autoclave (a pressure steam sterilizer), wrapped with gauze or paper, and placed either in a tray or in a glass tube. The pressure of the autoclave should be set at 30 pounds, the temperature at 270°F, and time at five minutes. Since the time to reach sterilization is about 20 minutes, and the drying time under vacuum is 20 minutes, the entire cycle lasts for approximately 45 minutes.

Skin needles with plastic handles are sterilized in a germicidal solution. Organic dirt, such as blood, plasma, feces, and tissue, absorbs the germicidal molecules and renders them inactive. The needles must be thoroughly washed with soap and water before immersion in germicidal solution.

A two percent aqueous alkaline solution of glutaraldehyde is claimed to be superior to alcohol. It has been reported to destroy all bacterial spores within three hours and tubercle bacilli within a few minutes. It is the liquid disinfectant of choice for instruments.

2. Disinfection of skin.[26,27] For hairy regions, a preliminary scrub with pHisoHex,® a synthetic detergent vehicle with three percent hexachlorophene, and water for five to ten minutes is indispensable. Tincture of iodine, a broad spectrum germicide against ordinary aerobic and anaerobic cutaneous bacteria and sporulating bacteria and fungi, may then be employed. This highly effective disinfectant has its drawbacks: Some patients are hypersenstive to it, and it leaves an unpleasant stain on skin and fabrics. Alcohol with concentration of between 70 and 92 percent can be used as a substitute. It destroys vegetative bacteria and tubercle bacilli promptly, although it is not effective against spores. It loses its "cidal" activity when concentration falls below 50 percent.

3. Disinfection of the acupuncturist's hands. Before starting the procedure, the acupuncturist must scrub his hands vigorously for five minutes and rinse with a solution of 75 percent alcohol for at least two to three minutes. If the fingers of his left hand are to be used to guide the needle, a rubber glove should be worn on that hand.

C. Body Postures

During acupuncture, the patient should assume a comfortable position and be able to maintain it for a long period of time. He must not move; otherwise the needle may bend or even snap off.[22]

The recumbent position is generally preferable. For acupuncture of points over the abdomen, face, and the anterior aspect of the extremities, the patient lies on his back (supine) with his knees supported. For acupuncture points over the back and the posterior aspect of the lower extremities, the patient lies on his stomach (prone) with his elbows propped. The lateral recumbent position may be satisfactory for acupuncture of points over the buttock area. A sitting position, with head and arms firmly supported, may be advised for acupuncture of points over the face and neck.

Since a patient experiencing acupuncture for the first time may become frightened or faint, the recumbent position must always be adopted for the initial attempt at this procedure.

D. Angle of Insertion

In general, there are three angles for insertion of the needle[22] (Fig. 5):

1. Straight insertion at a right angle to the skin. This is the most frequently-used approach for sensitive points located in regions where the musculature is relatively thick, such as over the upper and lower extremities. The potential danger of injuring blood vessels with this approach must be always borne in mind.

2. Bevel angle insertion at 45°. This approach is used in regions where musculature is relatively thin and vital organs lie relatively close to the skin, such as certain parts of the chest and back.

3. Reclining insertion at 12° to 15°. This approach is mainly used on the face. The needle penetrates the skin only and does not reach the muscle.

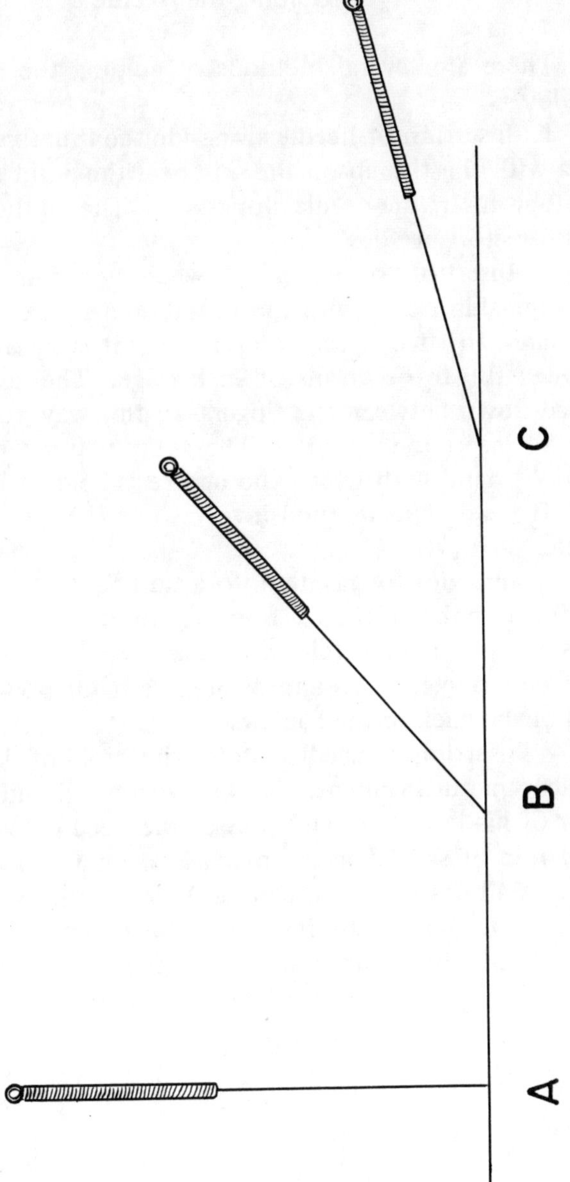

Fig. 5 Angles for insertion of needle. A. 90°. B. 45°. C. 12° to 15°.

E. Guiding the Needle

There are several methods of guiding the acupuncture needle:[22]

1. Insertion of needle alongside the thumbnail, (Fig. 6). Press with the thumb on the skin near the point of insertion, and then insert the needle alongside it. The method is usually used for short needles.

2. Insertion of needle between two fingers (Fig. 7). Press the skin down with the thumb and index finger of the left hand, in such a way that the point is situated halfway between the top sections of each finger. The needle is then guided down between the fingers. In this way, it is relatively easy to insert long needles. The acupuncturist can support the right hand with which the needle is held on the back of the left hand. This method involves less risk of breaking the needle.

3. Insertion of needle into a taut fold of skin (Fig. 8). Use the thumb and index finger of the left hand to stretch the skin into a taut fold with the point situated between these two fingers. This approach is used for points over the small of the back or the back itself.

4. Insertion of needle into a raised fold of skin (Fig. 9). The acupuncturist pinches the skin with the thumb and index finger of his left hand, and presses the needle down into the raised fold of skin. This approach is often used for points on the face and head where the musculature is relatively thin.

The needle can be inserted in several ways. It can, for instance, be simply jabbed in; it can also be rotated and "twirled" in. Regardless of the manner of insertion, the maneuver must be quickly and decisively done so that pain from penetration of the skin can be reduced to a minimum.

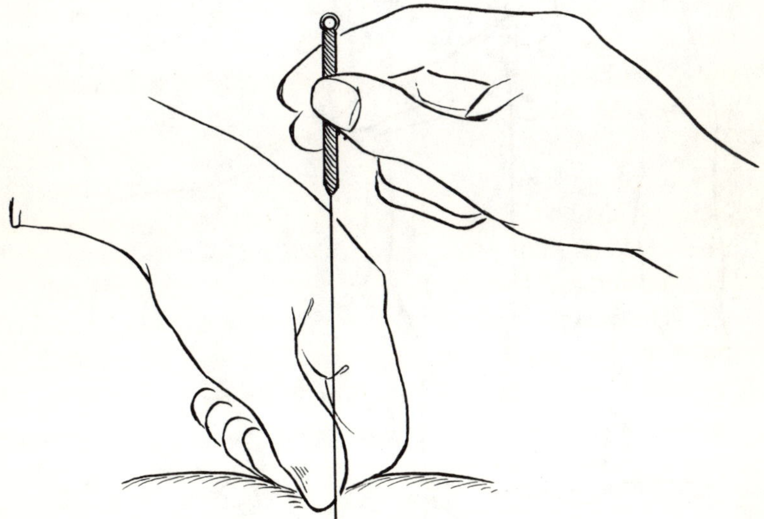

Fig. 6 Insert the needle alongside the thumbnail.

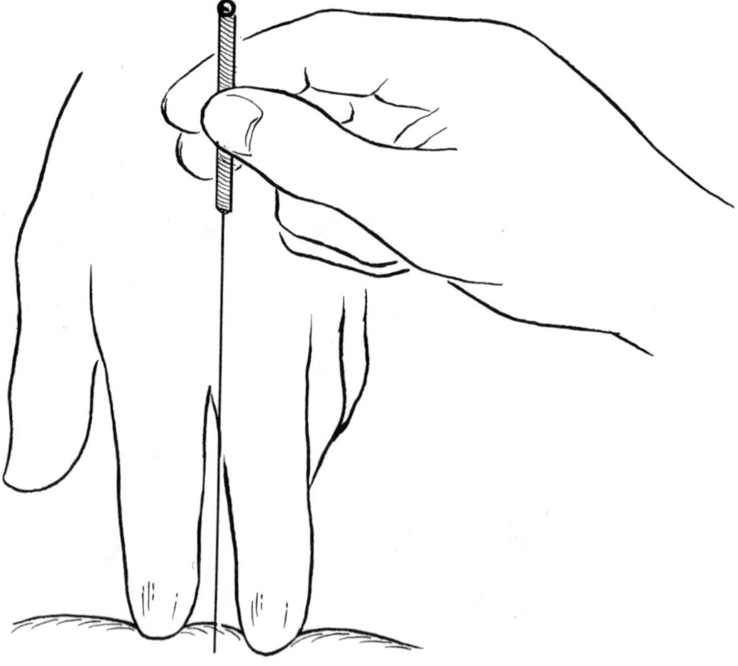

Fig. 7 Insert the needle between two fingers.

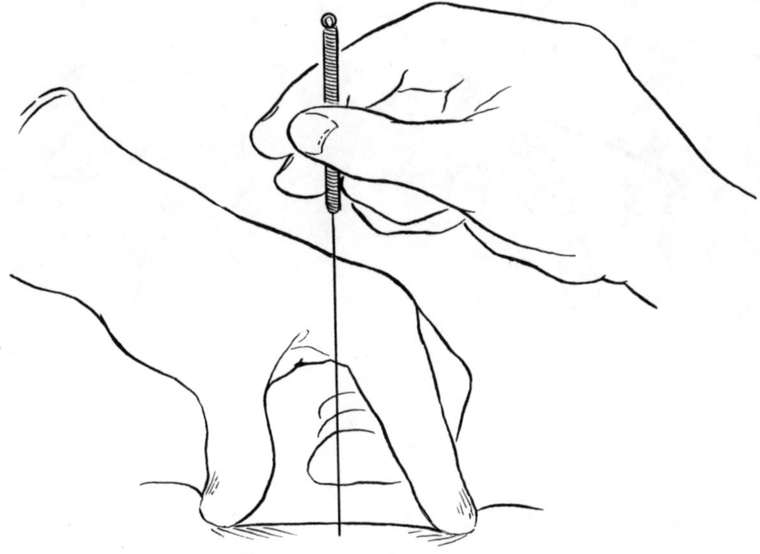

Fig. 8 Insert the needle into a taut fold of skin.

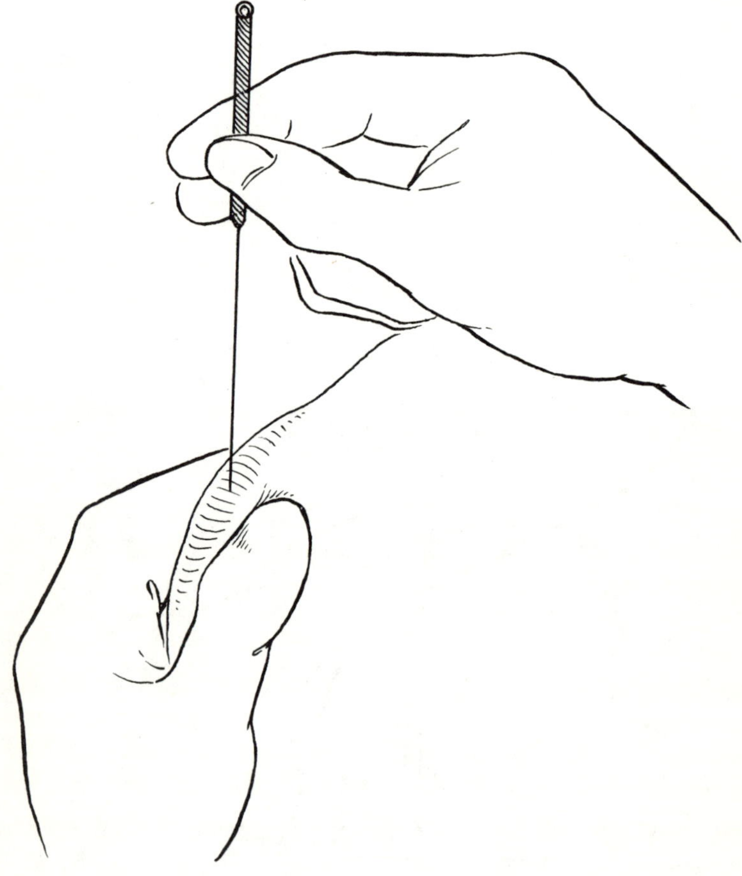

Fig. 9 Insert the needle into a raised fold of skin.

F. Sensations of "Take"

When the needle is inserted to a certain depth, the patient may experience a tingling sensation mixed with sensations of numbness, distention, and heaviness, classically known as the sensations of "take".[22,23] It is difficult to describe the sensations accurately, because they are somewhat different in each individual. Some patients describe the feeling as that of a fish being hooked, with the rod becoming suddenly heavy. Others says the tingling sensation is associated with propensity of distention and spreads to the distant periphery. The ancient books romantically suggest that a reaction occurs as if clouds are dispelled by a strong wind, and blue sky is suddenly visualized. All books have emphasized the importance of the sensation of "take." If this sensation promptly takes place, the effect of the acupuncture will be good. Without it, results are liable to be poor. Should the sensations of "take" not be obtained after insertion, an up and down rotation of the needle may promptly bring them out to light. If this is unsuccessful, another site should be chosen for acupuncture.

If after insertion of the needle, sensations of sharp pain instead of "take" are obtained, most likely the capillaries are punctured. The needle must be withdrawn and firm pressure applied to prevent bleeding.

Sometimes in addition to the sensations of pain experienced by the patient, fasciculations of the surrounding muscles may be observed. Sometimes fasciculations of the musculature may not be visible to the naked eye, but palpation of the region in the periphery of the acupuncture site may yield the tremulous sensation. The presence of fasciculations, visible or palpatory, indicates a good "take".[22,23]

G. Movement of the Needle

On many occasions, the sensation of "take" is not immediately experienced after the insertion of the needle. Special movements of the needle are necessary to bring about the sensation of "take"[23] (Fig. 10):

1. Rotation probing. After the needle is inserted to a certain depth, continuous rotation probing of the needle in the vicinity of the puncture may elicit the desired sensation.

2. Angle of rotation. Increasing the angle of rotation will increase the intensity of the stimulus. The stimulus may be further increased by gently pressing down on the needle. Generally speaking, the angle of rotation is between 90° and 300°, and the frequency of back and forth rotation[15] between thirty and forty times, although it can run as high as two hundred times per minute. If a weaker stimulation is desired, the operator may decrease the angle of rotation, and gently lift the needle a little. If a very strong stimulation is desired, the operator may rotate the needle continuously in one direction.

3. Stationary needle. When the needle is inserted to depth and the sensation of "take" is obtained by appropriate movement, the needle may be left in place for as long as two to three hours. The prolonged placement of the needle will increase the duration of the stimulus and reduce muscular spasm.

Physicians in ancient China followed complicated rules on the direction of the needle rotation in relation to the nature of disease, the synchronization of the needle insertion with exhalation and inhalation, and the time of the day during which the treatment should be given. Most of these rules are now nothing more than curiosities of medical history.

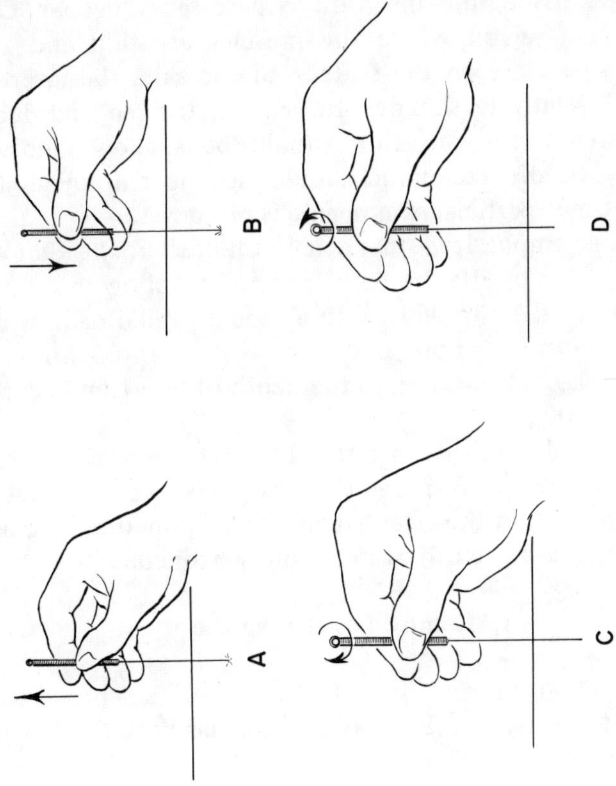

Fig. 10 Movement of the needle. A. Upward movement or partial withdrawal. B. Downward or probing movement. C. Clockwise rotation. D. Counterclockwise rotation.

H. Depth of Insertion

The depth of insertion depends upon the depth of sensory nerve endings or a sensory nerve.[22-23] In a region where the muscles are well developed and there is a quantity of adipose tissue, the insertion is necessarily deeper. Conversely, in a region where the muscles are thin and vital structures lie close to the surface of the skin, the insertion should be relatively shallow. In general, for old and debilitated patients, the insertion should be shallow, and the stationary needle technique should not be employed. For children, the superficial skin needle is preferred.

It was emphasized in ancient Chinese books that the insertion of the needle should be generally shallow in summer and relatively deep in winter. In a modern building in which the temperature is more or less consistent throughout the year, the seasonal variation in the depth of insertion becomes less important.

The usual depth of insertion is one to two centimeters. Rarely, a deeper set of nerve endings needs to be stimulated. The statement that the effectiveness of acupuncture increases with the increasing depth of insertion is erroneous.

I. Removal of the Needle

Special attention must be paid to the process of removing the needle.[22] Since the needle has been twirled and left in the tissue for a long period of time, its removal sometimes presents great problems. Ordinarily, the needle is gently rotated and withdrawn in two or three steps. The needle hole is then gently massaged with a piece of dry cotton or alcohol sponge. Occasionally, the needle is vigorously rotated, shaken, and quickly withdrawn in an attempt to increase the stimulation. This second method is now seldom used.

Sometimes it is impossible to remove the needle smoothly. This may be due to the following reasons: (1) change of position of the body whereby the needle becomes caught in the muscle mass; (2) bending of the shaft or tip of the needle as a result of vigorous twirling; (3) "hooking" of the needle on surrounding muscle or connective tissue fibers. The operator must not become panicky and try to pull the needle out by force. He must remain calm and rotate the needle gently and slowly until it is untangled from the surrounding structures. Sometimes in case of bending of the needle, the operator may have to maneuver the body of the patient to assume the original position. The needle can then be removed.

Sometimes acupuncture of a nearby site may be undertaken to relieve the muscular spasm and facilitate the removal of the needle. Sudden removal of the needle, without the above-mentioned precautions, causes further damage to the tissue and must be avoided.

J. Electric Stimulation

After a needle is inserted and the sensation of "take" experienced by the patient, electric stimulation may be applied.[25] There are many transistorized instruments available on the market, most of them powered by a six or nine volt battery (see Appendix II).

Electric stimulation is superior to manual stimulation, because its intensity can be easily regulated. During a prolonged operation, when anesthesia is required over a long span of time, it is indeed a labor-saving device. The voltage of the stimulating current should be increased to the maximum that the patient can tolerate or until slight fasciculations of surrounding muscle begin to appear. The duration of the stimulation should not be unduly prolonged lest adaptation of sensory nerves occur, and the "take" sensation diminish or disappear. During a lengthy operation, it is advisable to limit the stimulation to ten minutes at a time. Stimulation should be stopped for a few minutes and then resumed. Customarily, the needle is connected to the negative terminal of the stimulating unit, while a cotton ball, soaked with normal saline and applied to a distant region on the same side of the body, is connected to the positive terminal.

CHAPTER IV

TREATMENT OF COMPLICATIONS

Acupuncture, like other procedures, is not innocuous. Complications do arise occasionally and require special treatment.

(1) Vasovagal syncope or faint.[22,23,28] This complication occurs in patients who receive acupuncture treatment for the first time, those who are very apprehensive, the weak and debilitated, and those who react unfavorably to a strong stimulation. At first, the patient complains of dizziness, nausea, palpitation of the heart, and blurred vision. On examination, his face appears pale, blood pressure falls, and there is profuse perspiration. Later, he may become unconscious. The treatment for this condition is to remove all needles and to allow the patient to lie down, preferably with legs elevated. His airway must be kept open and his respiratory secretions suctioned out, if necessary. Warm drinks may be offered. Occasionally, in severe cases, atropine in large doses may be needed.

(2) Breakage of needle.[22,23] Occasionally, the needle is broken during acupuncture. There are many reasons for this complication: the needle may be weakened by rusting or erosion due to faulty storage; the body may be moved; the manual movement of the needle may be too vigorous. Should this happen, the operator must keep calm, keep the patient's position steady, and press down the skin on the sides of the needle. If the shaft of the needle is visualized, it can usually be removed by the use of forceps. Otherwise, the patient should be referred to a surgeon.

(3) Local reaction.[29] Sometimes because of vigorous movement of the needle, capillaries may be punctured and hematoma results, but it is usually not serious. Hot compresses may be applied to the site of hematoma. Pain and swelling usually subside in a day or two. It is theoretically possible that nerve injuries may occur in the process of acupuncture and the local area may feel numb for a few days. The feeling will gradually subside as the nerve regenerates from the injury.

(4) Infection.[29] If the aseptic techniques of the needles and the skin are strictly observed, local skin infection should not occur. Hepatitis is a dreadful possibility if the needles are not properly autoclaved. Disposable stainless steel needles packed in sterile plastic tubes may be a solution to this problem.

(5) Foreign body granuloma.[30,31] This rare complication occurred in the kidney parenchyma when the broken needle was left there for a long time.

(6) Cardiac tamponade.[32] One case was reported in literature when the needle had punctured the heart. It is evident that the acupuncturist must have a full knowledge of the anatomy of the body and must avoid using the needle deeply near the vital organs.

CHAPTER V

RECENT DEVELOPMENTS OF ACUPUNCTURE ANESTHESIA IN CHINA

Although acupuncture has been practiced for thousands of years in China, it was not until 1958 that the technique was officially introduced to the modern hospitals.[33] The adaptation of an old traditional method to aid the modern rigid disciplines of anesthesiology and surgery was not easy in the beginning. Only after many years of research, practice, and observation through the combined efforts of many health workers, did satisfactory results of anesthesia using acupuncture finally emerge. The important events of this worthy achievement may be summarized as follows:

A. Tonsillectomy

The first successful acupuncture anesthesia was used for tonsillectomy.[33,34] In the past, following tonsillectomy under local anesthesia, the patient usually complained of sore throat and inability to eat or drink for several days. Since acupuncture was noted to be very effective in relieving sore throat or pharyngitis, the question was posed as to why the procedure could not be used for postoperative sore throat. In practice it proved to be highly successful.[34] Often after one application of acupuncture following tonsillectomy, the patient stopped complaining of sore throat and was able to drink and eat happily. Acupuncture was later used as anesthesia for the tonsillectomy itself. Again, it was a success. The patient made much faster recovery after surgery. At present, almost all tonsillectomies in China are performed under acupuncture anesthesia.[33,34]

The most effective points for tonsillectomy have been found to be Ho-ku between two metacarpals of the hand, or Tzu-kou and Chih-cha over the forearm. (Chapter XIII, Fig. 11). The annoying gag reflex might be reduced by practicing with a tongue depressor in the throat before the operation.

B. Surgical Dressing

Acupuncture was also used before surgical cleansing of a wound. Ordinarily scrubbing or debridement of a wound causes the patient severe pain, and there is no effective local anesthesia that can be used. Acupuncture of a few proved points, such as Tsu-San-Li or Ho-ku greatly diminishes the intensity of pain arising from the surgical treatment of a wound.[34] It has been proved to be far superior to any known analgesic.

C. Comparison of Analgesic Potential of Points

The success of tonsillectomies and surgical treatment of a wound under acupuncture anesthesia gave rise to a number of experiments. First, using electronic pain-measuring instruments, the physicians in China compared the intensity of pain using acupuncture on themselves and on healthy volunteers. Based on the results of experiments conducted on more than 600 people, the analgesic potentials of 29 commonly-used acupuncture points were compared.[34] More than 40,000 experiments were done and data analyzed. These experiments proved without a doubt that different points differed greatly in their potentials for analgesic action and disproved the hypothesis that the more points of acupuncture stimulated, the better the therapeutic results. It was discovered that, in general, points with greater feeling of "take" produced better analgesic results. On the basis of these experiments, seven points were chosen for various operations.[34]

D. Induction Time

Experiments concerning induction time have been conducted on physicians in China. After stimulating the Fu-tu-point with electricity, the intensity of pain in the neck region was measured in relationship to time. The anesthetic effect of acupuncture reached its peak in twenty to thirty minutes.[35] Thereafter, the anesthetic effect did not further increase. Similar results have been observed in patients undergoing operations. Twenty to thirty minutes have to pass before the anesthetic effect is sufficiently strong to permit an operation.[35] The precise reason for the cumulative effect of acupuncture on the central nervous system is not known.

In a similar manner, with the application of electricity to the needle, the maximal anesthetic effect can be reached easily. Thereafter, increase of the electric potential even to the point that pain is produced will not augment the anesthetic effect.[35]

There is no appropriate explanation for the induction time. It is possible that the scene of the operating room creates a stress reaction in the patient with resultant increase of blood sugar, adrenaline output, blood pressure, and pulse. Such a stress reaction constitutes a rather unfavorable condition for acupuncture anesthesia. The surgeon must be patient and wait for the gradual return of the psychophysiological excitation to normal to insure good effects from acupuncture anesthesia. Preoperative administration of sedatives may reduce the excited state of the patient and render the induction time shorter. However, the part that stress plays is open to question. Calm patients still need an induction time of twenty to thirty minutes for the full development of anesthesia. The length of induction time does not seem to be directly related to the psychological state of the patient.[35]

E. Reduction of Acupuncture Points

When acupuncture anesthesia was still in its embryonic stage, it was thought that the more points stimulated, the more effective the results. During lung resection surgery, more than eighty needles used to be inserted into the four extremities of the patient, and four assistants had to be assigned to manually twirl the needles.[34] Later, after many experiments performed on the medical personnel themselves, only sixteen points on the upper and lower extremities on the side where the operation was performed were stimulated. The number of points stimulated was further reduced to twelve, and four years later – after many experiments and trials – to one, the Nei-kuan point on the arm. Using only the one point, the resultant anesthesia was even superior to the original custom of using more than eighty needles.[34]

Subsequently, an effort was made to reduce the number of points used for all operations. Experiments were carried out on more than 660 medical personnel and healthy volunteers, while prescriptions of acupuncture for more than 1,700 operations were analyzed and studied. More than 40,000 cases were collected and their data analyzed. Only 29 acupuncture points were ultimately selected for their relative effectiveness. The reduction of points was indeed a significant advance in acupuncture anesthesia.[34]

F. Treatment of Psychiatric Disease with Acupuncture

The success of acupuncture anesthesia has also inspired psychiatrists in China to search for new methods to treat psychiatric diseases.[36] Is it possible to transmit electricity through the sensory nerves to the higher center of the brain without affecting the motor cortex? This was the question posed by the Chinese psychiatrists.

There are three major types of treatment for severe psychiatric diseases in the Western countries.[36] The first is known as electric shock treatment. Two electrodes are placed on opposite sides of the patient's head and electricity is applied. Since the motor cortex of the cerebrum is stimulated, the patient undergoes violent generalized convulsions during the treatment. The second type is called insulin shock treatment. The blood sugar of the patient is artificially lowered by intravenous administration of insulin. The patient gradually lapses into coma with a very unpleasant experience. The third type is medicinal therapy with administration of large doses of tranquilizing or psychomotor drugs. The patient under such therapy is usually in a dull and nonproductive mental state.

The first problem encountered in experimenting with acupuncture for psychiatric use was the selection of points. In the beginning, according to the traditional Chinese methods, points over the four extremities were chosen for stimulation but the results were unsatisfactory. The Chinese psychiatrists then practiced acupuncture on themselves. They found that stimulation of points on their heads appeared to have a definite effect on their mental alertness. The same method was then used on patients. A case report described a markedly agitated patient who was readmitted to a psychiatric hospital.[36] He screamed, used obscene language, and destroyed practically everything within his reach, a totally unmanageable patient. During his previous hospitalizations, large doses of tranquilizers had to be given in addition to repeated electric shock treatments, but this time electric stimulation of acupuncture points on his head resulted in prompt disappearance of his symptoms. He was discharged after only a stay of half a month.

On another occasion, acupuncture treatment was given to a patient in a catatonic stupor. Contrary to the first patient, he lay in bed completely motionless. He did not eat, drink, or utter a single word. His dependence on others was total. In the past, the only treatment available to this type of patient was electric shock; however, the relapse rate was high. After electric stimulation of his acupuncture points was done a few times, the patient gradually recovered. Not only could he eat and drink normally, but he started to talk rationally.[36]

An outstanding characteristic of acupuncture treatment of psychiatric diseases is that the patient remains entirely conscious at all times. This cannot be achieved by means of electric shock, insulin shock, or tranquilizing drugs. Acupuncture is simple, convenient, and effective. There is no damage to the brain or other bodily structures.

Traditionally, psychiatric treatment aims at inhibition of the activities of the cerebrum. The physiological, as well as the pathological activities, of the cerebrum are suppressed. Acupuncture using electric stimulation seems to suppress the pathological activities only, and does not influence the physiological activities of the cerebrum at all. In the Shanghai Psychiatric Hospital, more than 1,200 patients have been treated, and approximately 73 percent have shown good to fair response.[36]

The mere fact that acupuncture using electric stimulation has a beneficial influence on psychiatric disease, indicates that it not only possesses an analgesic effect but also acts directly on the cerebral cortex. This observation indeed has added new insight as to the mechanism by which acupuncture works.

The treatment of psychiatric disease with acupuncture may sound incredible to the Western-trained psychiatrists.

However, in certain ways, the application of electro-acupuncture through the trigeminal nerve is analogous to the evolution of external to internal pacemaker for heart stimulation. In order to overcome the impedance of the skin and chest wall, the external pacemaker needs a current of 60 to 70 volts and causes annoying stimulation of many somatic muscles. The internal pacemaker, with tip of the electrode in the right ventricular cavity, needs a current of only one millivolt and does not stimulate any surrounding structure.

CHAPTER VI

THE NERVOUS SYSTEM IN ACUPUNCTURE ANESTHESIA

There is much evidence suggesting that the effect of acupuncture is mediated through the nervous system. The following observations were made by physicians after experimenting on themselves. Stimulation of the Ho-ku point caused the sensation of "take" and generalized anesthetic effect, more pronounced in the neck region.[34] Local infiltration of novocaine eliminated the sensation of "take" and the anesthetic effect. Application of a tourniquet to the upper arm until the artery became occluded within a certain period of time had no influence on the sensation of "take" and the anesthetic effect. These findings indicate that the nervous system, not the vascular system, is responsible for the acupuncture effect.[34]

A. Experiments with Novocain

The physicians in China further experimented on hemiplegic individuals.[37] The sensation of "take" could never be produced on the paralyzed side but could be immediately produced on the normal or unaffected side. They also experimented on patients who had received spinal anesthesia. Again, the sensation of "take" could not be produced in the lower extremities.

B. Experiments with Paraplegic Patients

During their study of the feelings of "take" the physicians soon learned that they were unable to produce the feelings in the lower extremities of a paraplegic individual even when points of proven greater sensitivity were stimulated.[37] Stimulation of points above the level of paraplegia immediately caused severe and prolonged feelings of "take." Later, they refuted their observation. In paraplegic patients with loss of deep and superficial sensation, but with preservation of the sweating function of the lower extremities, acupuncture of points below the level of paraplegia could still produce the feelings of "take." The preservation of the sweating function indicates that the sympathetic nervous system is still intact. For the paraplegic patients who had lost the ability to perspire, stimulation of the same points did not produce feelings of "take."[37] These observations served to indicate that the effects of acupuncture involve the autonomic nervous system as well as the somatic nervous system.

C. Neuroanatomical Dissection of Points

Neuroanatomical dissection of points was carried out on eight cadavers and 49 upper extremities and 24 lower extremities.[38] Needles were inserted by experienced acupuncturists into 324 points scattered throughout the body. The strict rules governing the angle and the depth of the insertion of the needle according to ancient literature were followed. It was indeed interesting to discover that there was definite nervous distribution under all points with the exception of Chu-ku (a point situated on the midline of the abdomen just above the symphysis pubis). Evidence of superficial nervous structure was found underneath 304 points, deep nervous structure in 170 points, and a combination of both superficial and deep nervous structure in 149 points. Further histologic examination of Chu-ku and 22 other selected points with the aid of differential stain revealed an abundance of nerve endings, sensory bodies, and even peripheral nerves at all depths from the skin down to deep muscles. It was postulated therefore, that the sensation of "take" following the stimulation with the needle depended upon the intactness of the nervous system.[38]

D. Direct Stimulation of Peripheral Nerves

As the effects of acupuncture had been demonstrated to mediate through the nervous system, the physicians in China began to ignore the acupuncture points and stimulate directly the areas rich in nerve endings, even the peripheral nerves. The result was just as satisfactory as stimulating the actual acupuncture points. First, the physicians experimented on themselves, an electrode being placed on a certain nerve in the neck and electricity applied. The cutaneous sensation in the neck gradually disappeared. Using the same technique, thyroidectomies were successfully performed under acupuncture anesthesia.[34]

It was further discovered that the closer the stimulus was applied to the site of operation, the better the anesthetic effect. It appears that if the afferent impulses from the acupuncture and the operation entered the same level of the central nervous system, the best anesthetic result would be achieved. Results after mechanical stimulation by twirling the needle and electrical stimulation were compared with both methods; the anesthetic effect was about the same.

E. Animal Experiments

Experiments were further carried out on cats.[34] An acupuncture needle was inserted into the lower end of the calf of a cat. A small bundle of nerve fibers was isolated from the main nerve in the leg and connected to a cathode ray oscillograph. Whenever the acupuncture needle was twirled, electric signals appeared on the fluorescent screen.[34] This suggests the theory that the sensation of "take" is conducted through the peripheral nerve. There may not be any visible nerve lying underneath the point, but the minute sensory bodies and nerve endings may produce the electric signals from the stimulation of acupuncture and send them to the peripheral nerve.

In another experiment,[34] painful stimuli were applied to the foreleg of a cat. At the same time, electric signals were recorded by a microelectrode implanted in a nerve cell located in the same segment of the spinal cord. The electric signals of the painful stimuli were greatly diminished or disappeared when an electric acupuncture needle was applied to the points or a peripheral nerve in the same leg. If the electric acupuncture needle was applied to the opposite leg, a reduction of the electric signal from the microelectrode could also be obtained.

These observations indicated that the transmission of nerve impulses in the spinal cord and brain not only occurred on the same side but also crossed the midline, at yet undefined levels, to reach pain reception centers on the opposite side. They led to the useful application of the acupuncture needle opposite to the site of the operation in procedures such as exploratory thoractomy and mitral commissurotomy. The convenience of administering acupuncture anesthesia was thus markedly increased.

CHAPTER VII

THE SYMPATHETIC NERVOUS SYSTEM IN ACUPUNCTURE ANESTHESIA

In regard to the relationship between the skin and the internal organs, the sympathetic nervous system plays a very important role.[39] In the previous chapters, it has been explained that the sensory impulses from the skin reach the spinal cord via the peripheral nerves. Since the internal organs are innervated by the sympathetic and parasympathetic nerves, which are in turn controlled by the cells located in the spinal cord, the electric potential of certain points may closely reflect the condition of certain internal organs. When the internal organ in question is diseased, the electric potential of the acupuncture points may be markedly altered. When the organ is removed, the electric potential of the point quickly returns to normal. For the same reason, one can understand why stimuli from acupuncture will influence the function of the internal organs, for example increasing their peristaltic activity.[39]

In the study of individuals with paraplegia due to spinal cord injury,[39] it was interesting to note that if the sympathetic fibers were intact, as evidenced by the presence of sweating in the lower extremities, stimulation of acupuncture points in the lower extremities could still easily induce the sensation of "take." But if there was no sweating, indicating damage to the sympathetic fibers, acupuncture in the lower extremities was not able to bring out any sensation of "take." In the latter instance, the findings resembled those seen in patients who were under spinal anesthesia.

A rabbit experiment is worth mentioning.[39] Stimulation of two points, the Ho-ku point on the foreleg and the Nei-ting point on the hindleg, greatly reduced the painful response of the nasal septum of the rabbit. But if the cervical sympathetic chain of the rabbit was severed, acupuncture of the same two points did not diminish the intensity of pain. In fact, it actually increased the intensity of pain. This experiment furnishes further evidence that acupuncture anesthesia mediates through the efferent limb sympathetic nervous system.

In still another experiment, the investigators in China cut the large sciatic nerve in the hindlegs of a dog.[39] Since pain is mostly transmitted through the sensory fibers of the sciatic nerve, the response to painful stimulation of the hindlegs of the dog was diminished. If the sympathetic nerve of the hindlegs of the dog was also cut, the response to painful stimulation increased. These findings indicate that the sympathetic nervous system probably exerts an inhibitory effect on the transmission of painful sensation through the cerebrospinal axis.[39] When the inhibitory effect is removed by the removal of the sympathetic nerve, more impulses of the painful sensation are transmitted to the center.

One hundred ten experiments were carried out on twenty rabbits to study the influence of acupuncture on peristalsis. Acupuncture of a point in the hindlegs of rabbits, corresponding to the Tsu-san-li point in humans, increased the peristaltic activity of the intestines. When all nerves in the periphery were cut, acupuncture still stimulated peristaltic activity. However, if the surrounding blood vessels were cut, acupuncture of the same point did not induce any peristaltic activity. If only the sympathetic nerve fibers were cut, while the blood vessels were left intact, acupuncture of the same point did not induce any peristaltic activity. The results of this procedure seem to indicate that the effects of acupuncture of that particular point in rabbits mediated through the sympathetic nerve fibers around the blood vessels.

Based on the above-mentioned observations, it seems highly possible that acupuncture excites the sympathetic nerve fibers around the blood vessels, which in turn send signals out to modify or block the transmission of painful sensation to the centers in the cerebral cortex.

CHAPTER VIII

ACUPUNCTURE OF THE TRIGEMINAL NERVE AND THE EAR

A. The Trigeminal Nerve

The trigeminal nerve is the largest cranial nerve, and its nucleus is the longest. It contains both motor and sensory fibers. The three sensory branches, ophthalmic, maxillary, and mandibular, supply all superficial sensation to the face and mucous membranes of the buccal cavity and eye. The sensory fibers of the gasserian or trigeminal ganglion enter partly into the reticular formation of the pons and partly into the cervical region of the spinal cord, as the descending or spinal trigeminal tract. The distribution of the trigeminal nerve is indeed widespread.

The concept of direct stimulation of the trigeminal nerve was conceived after repeated experiments on acupuncture anesthesia for appendectomy.[40] At first, based on ancient Chinese knowledge in acupuncture, four points on the face and nose were selected for stimulation. The results were fairly satisfactory. Later, the question was raised that since these four points were located in the distribution of the first and second branches of the trigeminal nerve, would it not be feasible to stimulate the branches directly and achieve the same therapeutic result. Experiments were again conducted on the physicians and the analgesic effects personally experienced. Then the technique was used as anesthesia for appendectomy, and it was a great success.[40]

The technique was later used for thyroidectomy, hernia repair, and brain, stomach, bladder, and kidney operations.

Hundreds of operations were performed with stimulation of the trigeminal nerve. Both surgeons and anesthesiologists were well satisfied with the results.[40]

Experiments were conducted on animals as well as humans.[40] Sensitive electronic instruments were attached to the brain and electric activity of the brain recorded. Stimulation of the trigeminal nerve elicited the strongest and widest distribution of the electric waves. Stimulation of other cranial nerves, on the other hand, induced much weaker electric waves of much smaller distribution. These findings served to explain the fact that stimulation of the trigeminal nerve produced a very satisfactory anesthetic effect for various operations over the entire body.

B. The Ear

It sounds incredible that acupuncture of the ear is an excellent anesthesia, but the fact is that since 1969, thousands of operations, covering any area from head to toe, have been performed in China under acupuncture anesthesia of the ear. The results have been acclaimed to be uniformly good.[41]

The following experiment was performed on Chinese physicians. Acupuncture needles were inserted into the Chiao-kan, Shen-men, Fei and Fu points of the ear (Fig. 11) (See appendix I for detailed description of points.) and mechanical stimulation applied in turn to each point for one minute.[41] Beginning with the fifth minute, needles were inserted into the abdominal wall at the frequency of one per minute. The purpose of inserting the abdominal needle was to elicit a uniform painful sensation for the volunteer physician to experience. The first abdominal needle caused clear-cut, and somewhat prolonged, pain. The tenth abdominal needle caused only dull pain of short duration. Thereafter, the painful sensation gradually disappeared. There was absolutely no pain from the fifteenth needle. Ten minutes later, with a total induction time of thirty minutes, all fifteen needles were removed without eliciting any pain. This experiment tended to demonstrate that the important principle in acupuncture anesthesia of the ear did not lie in the precise choice of points but in the proper induction time.

Recent neuroanatomical literature has indicated that there is an abundant nerve supply to the ear.[41] The ear is supplied by the sensory fibers of the trigeminal, facial, and vagus nerves of the cranial nerve system, and greater auricular (C_2 C_3) and greater and lesser occipital nerves (C_2) of the cervical spinal nerve system. The nerve endings are closely interwoven and superimposed on each other. Since these nerves have very wide distribution, stimulation of their branches in the ear has an analgesic effect on practically all parts of the body.

In another study checking senstive spots in the ear, it was found that in patients with duodenal ulcer, the stomach and duodenum points were quite sensitive to touch, whether by pinprick or by electronic instruments. During gastrectomy, these points seemed to extend to surrounding areas and become even more senstive to sensory stimuli. As the patient recovered from the operation, the sensitivity of these points gradually diminished. This observation appears to demonstrate the relationship between the sensitive points of the ear and the internal organs.

There were many interesting case reports describing the effectiveness of acupuncture anesthesia of the ear.[42] A woman with a twisted ovarian cyst was admitted because of excruciating abdominal pain. Insertion of needles into the ear reduced the pain promptly in a few minutes. A woman, ill, emaciated, and anemic with a huge ovarian carcinoma was operated on under "ear anesthesia." Although the operation lasted for over four hours, her blood pressure, pulse, and respiration remained stable.[42]

Thousands of operations have now been performed under "ear anesthesia" in China. The operations have been of all kinds – craniotomy, exploratory thoracotomy, gastrectomy, appendectomy, hysterectomy, and cataract removal. The results have been satisfactory.[42]

CHAPTER IX

SPECIFICITY AND NONSPECIFICITY OF ACUPUNCTURE ANESTHESIA

In ancient Chinese literature every point was regarded to be specifically effective for a certain disease. After many years of observation in modern China, however, considerable doubt has developed as to the validity of this hypothesis. For example, analysis of almost a thousand cases of tubal ligation performed in different hospitals revealed that there were many prescriptions given for acupuncture anesthesia.[43] Each prescription recommended different sets of points for stimulation. The results of all the various methods were quite satisfactory.

Based on this observation, it appears that for a given operation, many sets of points can be used with the desired comparable anesthetic effect. On the other hand, stimulation of one point may produce a generalized anesthetic effect throughout the body.

Studies were carried out to measure the anesthetic effect on different parts of the body when the Ho-ku point was stimulated. After an induction period, there developed different degrees of anesthetic effect over the various parts of the body, although the effect was most pronounced over the face. The fact that stimulation of the Ho-ku point caused a generalized effect illustrates the non-specificity of acupuncture anesthesia.[43]

In animal experiments, microelectrodes were inserted in the periphery of nerve cells located in the pain reception center of the thalamus. Electric waves were generated in the brain cells when a painful stimulus was applied to the body.

Electric waves were reduced in intensity or practically disappeared when an acupuncture point was simultaneously stimulated. The insertion of the needle into many different points of the upper and lower extremities produced varying reactions to the electric wave of the brain cell. It is known that nerve distribution is quite unequal throughout the body, some parts being very rich and some parts relatively poor in nerve supply. The more "effective" points seem to lie in the region where there is an abundant nerve supply.

Acupuncture anesthesia may exert its maximal effect in the same spinal segment. This was demonstrated by the following experiment: A painful stimulus was applied to the hindlimb of an animal. A microelectrode was inserted into the posterior horn of the same segment of spinal cord as the painful stimulus. A specific type of electro-physiologic wave could thus be obtained. The stimulation of a point located in the same segment would greatly diminish the amplitude of the electrophysiologic wave, while stimulation of points located in remote segments would have little effect on the electric wave.

In another experiment, a lower extremity of a monkey was artifically fractured. As expected sensitive spots began to develop on the monkey's ear. Slight pressure on the spots caused severe pain. Injection of local anesthetic into the lateral ventricles of the brain immediately abolished the sensitive spots. Destruction of other parts of the brain, however, had no effect on the existence of the sensitive spots on the ear. This experiment demonstrated the specificity of acupuncture anesthesia at the cerebral level.

The experimenters, therefore, concluded that there are two principles of acupuncture anesthesia – specificity and nonspecificity of points.[43] Studies must be undertaken to continue to search for points which have generalized or nonspecific effect on the entire body as well as points which have a localized or specific effect on certain operations.

CHAPTER X

ACTIVITIES OF THE RETICULAR FORMATION OF THE BRAIN STEM IN RELATIONSHIP TO ACUPUNCTURE ANESTHESIA

Although there is no definite proof, the activities of the reticular formation of the brain stem seem to play an important role in the effectiveness of acupuncture anesthesia.[44] The evidence supporting this hypothesis is as follows: (1) The effectiveness of acupuncture anesthesia depends to a certain degree on the mental state of the patient. The anesthesia will be effective if the patient is calm, cooperative, and confident about the procedure. The anesthesia will be less effective if the patient is agitated and overly concerned about the operation. However, if the patient is very drowsy or sleepy due to oversedation, the effectiveness of the acupuncture anesthesia will be nevertheless reduced. (2) The effectiveness of acupuncture anesthesia varies from individual to individual. Using the same acupuncture point, the same intensity of stimulation, the same induction time, and the same type of operation, the individual variation of effectiveness of the anesthesia is quite obvious. (3) Acupuncture may generate manifold regulatory effects on bodily functions such as on the blood pressure, pulse, respiration, and gastrointestinal motility. (4) Acupuncture of many different points in the body may produce the same anesthetic effect in certain operations and acupuncture of one certain point may produce anesthetic effect on many operations on the body.

Because of these facts, it is logical to assume that there

may be an important relationship between the reticular formation of the brain stem and acupuncture anesthesia.[44] According to recent neurophysiological studies, the reticular formation has widespread, diffuse, and non-specific effects. Two of the most prominent effects which have received considerable attention is the downstream influence upon the spinal cord and the peripheral motor system, and the upstream influence upon the cerebral cortex. The reticular formation also exercises regulatory control over many visceral and vascular activities. It can affect the respiratory rate, raise or lower the blood pressure, cause vasodilatation and vasoconstriction, and influence the function of the bladder. It affects also the basic physiological activities of the cerebral cortex such as sleep and alertness. Indeed, years of concerted study, both in man and in laboratory animals, will be required before this important and extremely complex mechanism is completely understood.

Experiments to study acupuncture effects on blood pressure were carried out on laboratory animals.[44] When the nerves of the animals were stimulated with a strong current, violent fluctuation in blood pressure ensued. Acupuncture rendered the fluctuation less or completely absent. If the nerve supplying the acupuncture point was cut, such an effect on the fluctuation in blood pressure disappeared. If the medulla oblongata was separated from the spinal cord, again the effect on the blood pressure disappeared. These experiments tend to indicate that the regulatory effect of acupuncture on blood pressure requires conduction above the spinal cord. When the peripheral nerve and the spinal cord were left intact, but the cerebral cortex was removed, the influence of acupuncture reached the brain stem. In such instances, the regulatory effect of acupuncture on blood pressure still existed. The last experiment tends further to demonstrate the importance of higher centers for the effect of acupuncture in altering the blood pressure.

In order to study further the relationship between the reticular formation of the brain stem and acupuncture anesthesia, experiments with therapeutic agents were carried out on laboratory animals. In 52 experiments on normal animals, anesthetic effects of various degrees were obtained 43 times, making the rate of effectiveness 82.7 percent.[44] The average induction time was 11 minutes, 30 seconds. The animals were then injected with many kinds of medicine which were known to have an effect on the central nervous system. Such medicines consisted of sedatives, hypnotics, analgesics, anesthetics, central stimulants, tranquilizers, antidepressants, psychotherapeutic agents, and autonomic drugs such as cholinergic and cholinergic-blocking agents, and adrenergic and adrenergic-blocking agents. The anesthetic effect of acupuncture was compared before and after the administration of these drugs. Some medicines evidently did increase the effectiveness of acupuncture anesthesia, but some invariably reduced it. For example, barbiturates with their analgesic and sedative effect, seemed to work against acupuncture and reduce its effectiveness. Some medicines, although without any analgesic action, definitely increased the effectiveness of acupuncture anesthesia. It was most interesting to observe that some central stimulants could actually potentiate the effectiveness of acupuncture anesthesia. These findings further support the hypothesis that acupuncture anesthesia can be influenced by the functional state of the central nervous system and is not effective simply due to suppression.

Recent pharmacological studies have demonstrated that the principal action of the drugs which increase or decrease the effectiveness of acupuncture anesthesia is on the reticular formation of the brain stem. For example, the effects of anesthetic and sedative drugs mediate through the inhibition or blockage of activities of the reticular formation of the brain stem. The stimulants used in the experiments had effects on the cerebral cortex, spinal cord, or on the brain stem. Only the group of stimulants whose pharmacological action was on the brain stem increased the effectiveness of acupuncture anesthesia. Evidently the effectiveness of acupuncture anesthesia was increased when the functions of the reticular formation of the brain stem were stimulated, and decreased when the latter functions were suppressed. Pharmacological effects on acupuncture may indeed open a new method for investigation of the reticular formation of the brain stem.[44]

CHAPTER XI

THE ANATOMY AND PHYSIOLOGY OF PAIN WITH PARTICULAR REFERENCE TO ACUPUNCTURE ANESTHESIA

Wolff and Wolff began in their famous monograph, "pain",[45] by saying, "Pain is one of Man's major concerns. Probably more than any other symptom pain is responsible for bringing the patient to the doctor. Thus to the clinician the understanding of pain becomes a paramount concern. Despite the importance of pain in diagnosis and the challenge it offers in therapy, however, the doctor has no certain way of knowing how much pain his patient is experiencing. As in the case of other sensations, he knows of the pain only through the patient's testimony."

Perhaps because of this difficulty, although extensive investigations have been carried out in the last two decades, very little is yet known of either the anatomical or the physiological mechanisms subserving this mode of sensation. More investigations are evidently needed, and results from empirical use of acupuncture may indeed provide new impetus to its understanding.

Our current concept of pain reception has undergone quite a radical change. For a long time, the histologists had been enchanted by such connective tissue capsules such as Meissner's tactile corpuscles, spherical end-bulbs of Krause, Golgi-Mazzoni corpuscles, and Vater-Pacinian corpuscles in the subcutaneous tissue.[46,47] They were thought to be responsible for the different qualities of sensation, such as warmth, cold, touch, light, and pain. In other words, it was thought that the sensation depended largely on the type of receptor which was stimulated rather than the character of the stimulus. However, subsequent studies have proved that this theory of "Receptor Specificity" is erroneous. Pain reception actually depends upon the free nerve endings. In cornea, tooth pulp, and tympanic membrane where only free nerve endings are present, all sensations of touch, warmth, cold, and so on can be appreciated. Furthermore, it has been found that the free nerve endings are distributed everywhere in the body from which pain may be perceived, and in some of these sites, they are the only receptors present.[46, 47] From these endings, sensory impulses are carried through the myelinated and unmyelinated fibers of various sizes to the posterior root ganglia or the corresponding ganglia in the head. Some sensory impulses are carried through the sympathetic trunks and through the sympathetic ganglia to the posterior root ganglia via the white rami communications.

The sensory nerve fibers have been classified according to their sizes as well as according to the speed that they conduct impulses. The small fibers conduct impulses slowly and the large fibers conduct them more rapidly. For example, the large A-delta myelinated fibers have diameters from 10 to 20 microns and are able to conduct impulses up to 30 meters per second. The small C unmyelinated fibers have diameters about 3 microns and conduct impulses one to two meters per second. There is some evidence to suggest that the painful sensation is transmitted through the small C fibers, while non-painful sensation, such as from acupuncture, is transmitted through the large A fibers.[48] However, such a hypothesis must be viewed with extreme caution because in controlled physiological studies, it is difficult to demonstrate different pain qualities in normal subjects using electric stimuli, and there are many A and C fibers conducting all modalities of sensation, including pain.[49] Nevertheless, it may be safe to say that there are A and C fibers which respond to certain stimuli and not others. In other words, these fibers are modality-specific.[50]

The cell bodies of all sensory nerves lie in the posterior root ganglia. From there, the dendrites of neurons which subserve pain may either ascend or descend one or two segments in the zone of Lissauer before reaching the spinal cord. Anatomical data based on painstaking dissection of the spinal cord suggest that all these primary afferents ultimately terminate in the substantia gelatinosa.

In the gate-control theory of Melzack and Wall, the cells in the substantia gelatinosa play a central role in controlling the pain inputs to the higher centers. This theory[52] suggests that the SG cells presynaptically inhibit or modulate all impulses from the afferent cutaneous fibers. The painful impulses transmitted in the small diameter fibers inhibit the SG cells and travel to the transmission cells in the spinal cord. The impulses transmitted in the large diameter fibers excite the SG cells and further inhibit the transmission of painful stimuli to the higher centers. The important point in this theory is that impulses transmitted in the large diameter fibers may inhibit impulses in the small diameter fibers. Furthermore, the psychological function of the individual may modulate the activity of the SG cells and influence the transmission of sensory impulses.[53]

There are many examples of this theory. The common practices of massage, pressure, vibration, cold and hot compresses are known to alleviate the sensation of deep pain to a large extent. The technique of using an ethyl chloride spray before minor surgery on the skin is another example. Selective stimulation of the large diameter fibers with minimal electric current has been proved effective in many instances of chronic pain syndrome. Indeed, this is the principle used in electroanalgesia by dorsal column or peripheral nerve stimulation. Very possibly this may also be the principle in acupuncture anesthesia. The familiar example of an athlete with severe knee injury who does not complain much during the heat of the game demonstrates how psychology influences pain appreciation.

However, recent experiments indicate that the detailed neuronal circuitry of the gate-control model may be incorrect.[54] The gate-control theory predicts that after the activation of the pain fibers, the SG cells would be inhibited and the excitability of the primary afferent fibers would be decreased. In reality, electrical stimulation of substantia gelatinosa during application of a painful stimulus in the periphery increases, rather than decreases, the excitability of the afferent fibers. But one word must be added: Despite challenges to the detailed neuronal circuitry in the spinal cord, the basic contention of the gate-control theory stands. This theory does explain many neurophysiological phenomena which have been heretofore unexplainable. However, exactly where the block in the central nervous system is located remains a question.

After modulation by the SG cells, the sensory impulses then switch to a second neuron whose cell body lies in the posterior horn from which the impulses are promptly transferred either directly or through additional neurons to the opposite side of the spinal cord via the anterior commissure.[51, 53] Without further synapses, the impulses travel in the lateral spinothalamic tract to the thalamus. There is evidence, however, that some fibers ascend on the ipsilateral side and do not cross at all and that the fibers associated with pain are situated anteriorly while those associated with temperature are situated posteriorly in the tract. Despite the large number of investigations which have been performed, the precise anatomical and physiological organization of the spinothalamic tract remains somewhat unclear.

The fibers in the spinothalamic tract give off branches to the reticular formation along the way. Impulses going into the reticular formation are thought to provide the mechanism responsible for consciousness and to supply electrical energy to many brain circuits. Again, the functional significance of the spinothalamic projection to the reticular formation is poorly understood.

In the thalamus, the impulses are transferred to additional neurons which are located in the thalamico-cortical radiation. Although specific sites in the cerebral cortex responsible for pain appreciation are not known, anatomical evidence suggests that fibers from the posterior thalamus project directly to the secondary sensory area (somatic area II). When the sensory impulses reach the higher centers in the cerebral cortex, they are naturally subjected to interpretation, followed by formulation of the individual's reaction toward them.

Most of the sensory impulses from the head region are carried in the trigeminal nerve through its three branches.[51] The first or ophthalmic branch leaves the cranial cavity through the superior orbital fissure, and supplies the sensation to the lacrimal gland, conjunctiva, mucous membrane of the upper nasal cavity, part of the skin of the nose, the upper eyelid, the forehead, and the anterior part of the scalp. The second or maxillary branch reaches the face through the infraorbital canal. It supplies the maxillary sinus, upper teeth, cheek, uper lip, and nose. The third or mandibular branch leaves the skull through the foramen ovale. It supplies the chin, and the mucous membranes of the lower jaw.

The cell bodies of these three sensory branches of the trigeminal nerve are located in the gasserian ganglion on the anterior surface of the tip of the petrous bone. The central processes of these cells enter the middle part of the pons in two groups. One group enters the main sensory nucleus in the lateral pontine area. Fibers from this nucleus cross in the reticular formation to the opposite side and ascend with the medial lemniscus to the thalamus. The other group descends into the cervical region of the spinal cord as the descending or spinal trigeminal tract.

It is interesting to note that in some respects, the trigeminal system resembles the spinothalamic system. The three sensory branches of the trigeminal nerve are comparable to the somatic nerves, the gasserian ganglion to the posterior root ganglion, and the spinal trigeminal tract to the fibers of the posterior horn of the spinal cord. Although the gate-control mechanism has been only demonstrated in the spinal cord, it is highly conceivable that a similar mechanism may be operating in the trigeminal system, as well. Furthermore, since the trigeminal system lies in closer proximity to the central nervous system than the spinothalamic tract, the impulses reached by this system may exert a relatively stronger influence on the higher centers in the cerebral cortex. Of course, this is just speculation. However, the results of using facial needles for major operations and facial massage preceding dental extractions in China tend to support this hypothesis.

CHAPTER XII

CURRENT CONCEPTS OF ELECTROANALGESIA

Entirely separate from the development of acupuncture in China, concepts of electroanalgesia have gradually evolved in the United States in recent years. The technique, however, has never been used as an attempt to induce anesthesia for surgery, but rather as a method to achieve prolonged relief of pain in patients with chronic pain syndrome.

The patients who suffer from chronic pain syndrome include those with metastatic cancer, nerve injuries, amputations with phantom limb syndrome, paraplegia with pain of the extremities, lumbar disc surgery, and causalgias. These patients are first treated with increasing doses of analgesic and narcotic medications, and when their pains persist, such neurosurgical procedures as percutaneous spinal cordotomy, rhizotomy, spinal commissurotomy, tractomy, or sympathectomy are tried. Only after all these measures fail to relieve their pain, are they finally given a trial with electroanalgesia.

Success with electroanalgesia was first reported on stimulation of peripheral nerves. Wall and Sweet[55] in 1967 reported successful treatment of eight patients with severe cutaneous pain by stimulation of their peripheral nerves. Total anesthesia of the skin area supplied by the nerve was achieved. Following stimulation, four patients continued to experience anesthetic effects for more than 30 minutes, and four patients reported a return of their skin sensation within a few seconds to a few minutes. Sweet and Wepsic[56] in 1968 reported success in some of their eighteen patients with chronic intermittent peripheral stimulation. In their study, electrodes were implanted in the vicinity of the peripheral nerves and then activated by external radiotransmitters.[57]

In 1969, Shealy and his co-workers[58] offered for the first time a detailed description of dorsal column stimulation in patients with chronic pain syndrome. They believed that careful selection of patients was of key importance in assuring the success of the procedure. In their view, a psychiatrist, trained and interested in pain patients, should be an intimate part of the team effort neeeded to manage such patients. The Minnesota Multiphasic Personality Inventory was used as an aid in patient selection. It was felt that patients with more than four personality traits elevated over two standard deviation should be operated on only with great caution, while elevations of depression, hysteria, and hypochrondriasis scales do not preclude surgery.

They believed also that some form of trial electrical stimulation is essential for the selection of patients because occasional patients[59] may object to the sensation of buzzing. Skin electrodes were applied at different sites and a tingling sensation was induced in the areas of pain. This led to some degree of pain relief and allowed the patient to decide the value or possible annoyance of electrical stimulation. If there were any questions concerning the patient's response to transcutaneous electrical stimulation, the percutaneous technique of dorsal column stimulation by Hosobuchi, Adams, and Weinstein[60] would be used. In that case, a 22-gauge needle was introduced into the C1-C2 interspace (ipsilateral to the painful area) under radiographic control. A myelogram was done with 1 cc of cerebrospinal fluid emulsified with pantopaque to delineate the dentate ligament. The needle was then withdrawn and reinserted 3 to 4 mm dorsal to the ligament. A 10-mil electrode was introduced into the cord through the needle and the dorsal column was stimulated at different depths and with different voltages, frequencies, and duration of electric current. If the sensation from the percutaneous stimulation was pleasurable, or unpleasant but tolerable, and relief of pain was good, surgery for permanent implantation with an electrode could then be considered.

Based on clinical evaluation, Shealy[58, 59] reported that it was best to place the electrode four to six spinal segments above the highest pain input. For arm pain, the electrode was placed at C2 to C4, for chest or abdominal pain at D2, and for pelvic or leg pain at D2 to D4 or D6 to D8. Because the procedure involves the insertion of a foreign body near the arachnoid and exposure to the cerebrospinal fluid, antibiotic treatment using methicillin or sodium cephalothin by intravenous drip was advised during the operation and for a few days after.

The neurosurgical procedure involving actual implantation of the electrode and radioreceiver is as follows: A standard bilateral laminectomy is performed, making certain that the exposure of the dura mater is adequate to accept the electrode. In most cases, two or three spinous processes and one set of lamina are removed. A 3-inch transverse incision is made, centered over the clavicle, for the placement of the receiver. A subcutaneous tunnel through the paraspinal muscles is developed by blunt dissection from the incision over the shoulder to the laminectomy site. A small subcutaneous pocket just large enough to accomodate the receiver is developed below the lower flap of the clavicular incision. The dura is then carefully opened with a midline incision. A pocket, large enough to accomodate the electrode is dissected beneath the dura. The electrode is a platinum plate of about 5 mm square attached on a piece of silicone-impregnated, dacron which is anchored to the dura with No. 4-0 nonabsorbable sutures. Needless to say, the placement of the electrode must be precise and requires the skills of a neurosurgeon well acquainted with the procedure.

The electric stimulus is delivered to the implanted radio-receiver transcutaneously from an external battery-powered radio-transmitter.

Pulse widths of 0.3 msec with repetition rates ranging from 50 to 275 pulses per second are available to the patient and under his control. The intensity of voltage delivered is similarly controllable by the patient. In a brief experimental run with an alternative external stimulator, a varity of pulse shapes are used, including sine, triangular, round, and square biphasic waves. All patients seem to like the square biphasic waves for best response. Patients also seem to prefer a pulse rate between 100 and 200 per second.

Voltages vary from 0.3 to 3.0 volts, the higher level being used only with monopolar electrodes. With a bipolar arrangement, less than 0.5 volts is adequate for stimulation. This current, measured in one patient with a special receiver, was approximately 0.5 mA. With the large surface area of the electrode, the total power density was well below 0.05 W/in^2, the level for threshold damage in experimental studies.

In response to dorsal column stimulation, all patients in the Shealy experiments experienced a buzzing or tingling sensation radiating from the site of the stimulator down the spinal cord and along the sciatic nerves to the feet. Some relief of pain was achieved in all patients. Patients usually experienced great relief of pain only while the dorsal columns were stimulated. One patient found that after three or four hours of stimulation, she became bored or annoyed by the presence of stimulation and turned it off. Her pain of course promptly returned. There was no lasting benefit from stimulation. The pain threshold in all patients as measured by Noterman's technique of skin stimulation[61, 62] was raised from 50% to 250% over base levels during dorsal column stimulation. Return to the prestimulation threshold occurred promptly after cessation of dorsal column stimulation.

The patients had no difficulty in walking during the dorsal column stimulation. Muscle power, motor function bladder and bowel control, erection, and ejaculation were not altered. Touch, position, and vibratory sensation were intact. A pinprick was reported to lead to a slightly hyperalgesic response in the skin of the legs, but deep pressure was less painful than normal.[63, 64]

The success of dorsal column stimulation led to trancutaneous stimulation of peripheral nerves in patients with causalgia.[65] At the Walter Reed General Hospital, patients with pain secondary to nerve injury and who had obtained incomplete relief from non-narcotic analgesics were referred for study. An accessible site, central to the point of injury was selected for stimulation. The stimulation parameters were similar to those described for dorsal column stimulation – 0.1 msec duration, unidirectional square pulses of variable voltage and a rate of 100 per second. Electrodes consisted of insulated stiff copper wires, tipped with stainless steel balls of 3 mm diameter and 2 cm separation. They were moistened with electrolyte paste and applied directly over the course of the nerve trunk being stimulated. A series of eight patients with causalgia was studied. Immediate dramatic relief of pain was obtained in six patients during stimulation and for variable durations up to seven hours even after stimulation was ended.

There seems no doubt that electroanalgesia was effective in patients who suffered from chronic pain syndrome.[66] Although the analgesic effect might be only partial, it did offer the only hope to sufferers after all other measures had failed. How long the dorsal column or the peripheral nerves can be stimulated without losing the analgesic effect and without causing permanent damage remains a matter to be decided through further observation.

CHAPTER XIII

THE SELECTION OF ACUPUNCTURE POINTS

Combining the disciplines of traditional Chinese medicine and modern concepts of neuroanatomy and neurophysiology, anesthesiologists in China have selected a number of points for surgical anesthesia. These points have been repeatedly used on thousands of patients over a period of many years. They have been found to be relatively more effective. Sometimes one point is used for many operations, and sometimes many points are used for one operation. The selection of points is by no means final because continuous research is being carried out to further increase the effectiveness of acupuncture anesthesia. Occasionally, the standard surgical procedures have to be modified to ensure tolerance and comfort of the patients. Their experience in selecting points for a few representative operations is summarized as follows: (Fig. 11) (See appendix I for detailed description of points.)

A. Dental Extractions

More than 5,000 dental extractions have been performed under acupuncture anesthesia. It was reported that 80.8% of patients experienced no pain, 16.9% mild pain, and 2.3% relatively severe pain.

The needle is usually inserted to point 35 at a 30 to 45 degree angle, and then advanced to point 7. The local acupuncture on the same side is performed later. The tip of the needle is directed toward the diseased tooth.

	Distant points on the opposite side	**Local points on the same side**
Upper incisor	Point 35 through 7	Points 43 and 42
Lower Incisor	Same as above	Points 44 and 39
Upper canine	Same as above	Points 43 through 42 and 41
Lower canine	Same as above	Points 44 through 40 and 39
Upper premolar	Same as above	Points 38 and 41
Lower premolar	Same as above	Points 44 and 39
Upper molar	Same as above	Points 41 and 39
Lower molar	Same as above	Points 44, 39 and 38

When the patient complains of pain and becomes very apprehensive, or when the oral surgery is of relatively long duration, acupuncture of the point 34 on the ear is used. For patients who are extremely nervous and who have hypertension, points 26 and 32 on the ear are sometimes used.

After the sensation of "take" is obtained, the needles are twirled for one to two minutes. The needles are then left in place for one to five minutes and twirled again for one to two minutes. Dental surgery is carried out afterwards. Customarily the needles are left in place during the operation. However, if placement of the needle interferes with the proposed surgery, it may be removed. After the operation, the local and the ear needles are removed first. The needle in point 35 is usually kept there for at least five minutes longer to ensure satisfactory analgesia.[67-69]

B. Thyroidectomy

More than 400 thyroidectomies have been performed under acupuncture anesthesia. Good result was obtained in 86.5 percent and fair result in 13.5 percent.

Point 9 (Fu-tu) seems to be the best point for thyroidectomy. A needle of 1.5 inches in length is inserted to that point on both sides. The direction of the needle is parallel to the posterior margin of the sternocleidomastoid muscle. Another needle of the same length is inserted 0.5 cm posterior to point 9 and parallel to the first needle. This needle serves as the indifferent electrode. These two pairs of needles are then connected to two electric stimulating instruments and stimulated with the maximal intensity of electricity that the patient can tolerate.

C. Tonsillectomy

A few thousand tonsillectomies have been performed under acupuncture anesthesia. The following three points were reported to be most effective: (1) Point 7 (Ho-ku) on both sides; (2) Point 36 (Tzu-kou) on both sides; and (3) Point 37 (Chih-cha) on both sides. Generally speaking, electric stimulation of the needle is preferable.

The only drawback with this operation is that when the pharynx is in contact with surgical instruments or blood, the gag reflex remains present after acupuncture anesthesia. The gag reflex may be reduced to the tolerable degree by asking the patient to practice with a tongue depressor in his throat the day before planned surgery.[70–72]

D. Pulmonary Surgery

In the beginning, approximately a hundred needles were employed for a case of pulmonary resection. After many years of research and trial, the ineffective points were systematically eliminated. Successful anesthesia may now be obtained by the use of only one needle to stimulate only one point. There are three points found to be most effective for this purpose: (1) Point 3 (Nei-kuan), with deep penetration

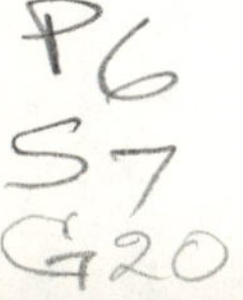

0.5 to 1.5 inches; (2) Ting-hui point, slightly inferior and posterior to point 38 (Hsia-kuan), obtained with mouth open; and (3) Point 45 (Feng-chih) on the same side with the operation, using a four or five-inch long needle.

Precautions: (1) In order to prevent mediastinal flutter and substernal pressure feeling during operation, the patient usually has had breathing exercises for the few days prior to the operation. The best result is seen in patients who are able to breath only six or eight times a minute for as long as half an hour. (2) The anterior axillary incision is adopted because the patient may lie on his back during the operation. Since there is less musculature in that region, opening the chest wall in that region will take less time. (3) Intercostal nerve block with one percent procaine is frequently used to reduce pain from skin incision and rib resection. (4) In the pleural cavity, the surgeon usually avoids touching the lung or diaphragm with his fingers. When the bronchi are manipulated, the patient is instructed to have deep breathing with his mouth open. In this way the cough reflex may be minimized. Sometimes, injection of 0.25 percent procaine in the periphery of bronchi may block the cough reflex. (5) Because the analgesia is usually not complete, the placement of the drainage tube and suturing up the skin must be accomplished in the shortest time possible. (6) For patients with large amounts of expectoration and very poor pulmonary function, endotracheal intubation is desirable. Even with acupuncture anesthesia, preliminary spray with some anesthetic agent in the throat is often necessary for intubation.[73]

E. Gastric Surgery

Patients with gastric or duodenal ulcers, pyloric obstruction, hemorrhage, gastric performation, or carcinoma are candidates for acupuncture anesthesia. Types of gastric surgery consist of subtotal or total gastrectomy, pyloroplasty with vagotomy, and gastrojejunostomy.

The points used for this operation are point 19 (Tsu-san-li) and point 21 (Shang-chu-hsu) on both sides or on the left side. Most of the patients experience practically no pain or distension, nausea, vomiting, or urinary retention after surgery. They are able to resume ambulatory activities two days after operation, drink liquids on the fifth day, and enjoy a normal diet in one week.

However, the anesthesia is not without its disadvantages. First, the analgesic effect is not complete, especially when the peritoneum is touched. Secondly, the patient may experience some discomfort when the internal organs are manipulated. The discomfort is sometimes quite severe during ligation of gastric artery, exploration for disease in the duodenal bulb, or lysis of surrounding adhesions. Thirdly, there may be incomplete relaxation of abdominal muscles.

F. Appendectomy

Some anesthesiologists prefer point 7 (Ho-ku) or point 3 (Nei-kuan) on the right arm, while the others prefer point 21 (Shang-chu-hsu), point 19 (Tsu-san-li), point 24 (Yai-chung) or point 23 (San-yang-chiao).

G. Herniorrhaphy

Point 23 (San-yang-chiao) and point 21 (Shang-chu-hsu) are usually used.

H. Tubal Ligation

Face needles or stimulation of the trigeminal nerve are usually used.

I. Knee Operation

In this operation, the choice of points is based on the distribution of peripheral nerves rather than traditional Chinese medicine. Needles are inserted just below the lateral third of the spinous processes of the third and the fourth lumbar vertebra, and electrical stimulation applied. The skin around the knee joint feels thickened and numb. It offers no sensation with pinpricking. Since joint is supplied by deep nerves also, stimulation of the following nerves yields almost perfect anesthesia: (1) Femoral nerve (lateral to the pulsation of femoral artery in the inguinal region, about 3.5 inches lateral to the symphysis pubis); (2) Ischial nerve (1.5 inches above the center of gluteal fold) and (3) Lateral cutaneous nerve of thigh (Point 18, depressed area below the anterior margin of head of fibula).

CHAPTER XIV

PSYCHOLOGICAL PREPARATION OF THE PATIENT

In the practice of acupuncture anesthesia, it has been observed that some operations always produce good results and the patients are generally very well satisfied, whereas some operations often do not produce good results with a majority of the patients left somewhat dissatisfied. Why is there such a difference in the performance of the operators? Because the points are poorly chosen? No. Because there is no "take" after acupuncture? No. The difficulty lies in the personal relations between the patients and the operators.

It would be a mistake to assume that acupuncture consists simply of twirling a needle. Some health workers, after watching a few acupuncture demonstrations think that the procedure is extremely simple, requiring nothing more than a few rotations of the needle. When they return to their home stations and have the opportunity to practice on their own patients, their efforts result in failure! They blame the logic of acupuncture! This is an extremely poor way to learn how to utilize acupuncture as a means of anesthesia.

One basic principle underlying acupuncture anesthesia is that the patient remains totally conscious through the entire operation. Except for the fact that the sensation of pain diminishes or disappears, all sensations remain intact. The patient lying on the operating table is aware of his surroundings and hears every sound in the operating room. Not infrequently, he feels the pulling and pushing of his viscera and other sensations related to the operation. Under such circumstances, it is not difficult to appreciate the importance of the psychological preparation of the patient. Experience has shown that patients who have had no knowledge of an operation beforehand become extremely apprehensive and fearful in the operating room. They cannot cooperate fully with the surrounding anesthesiologists and surgeons. The results of acupuncture anesthesia in those circumstances are, of course, unsatisfactory. Not infrequently in such cases, during the course of the operation, acupuncture anesthesia has to be terminated and conventional anesthesia with pharmacological agents used. These fearful patients are considered by some health workers to be uncooperative. But are these patients really uncooperative?

To the patient an operation constitutes a major event in his life. It is entirely understandable that the patient does not comprehend the nature of the operation and becomes unduly worried and apprehensive during the procedure. Health workers must appreciate the psychology of the patient and spend time explaining the nature and necessity of an operation. They must describe what sensations the patient may experience during surgery. Until the surgeons and anesthesiologists have won the confidence of the patient, no operation should be contemplated.

In China, health workers practice acupuncture first on themselves, experiencing the sensation of "take." Searching for more effective points, they have had to insert as many as forty needles into their bodies at one time. The experience they gained served an immensely useful purpose in later counseling and comforting patients. It is their slogan that "they must see as their patients see, feel as their patients feel, and work entirely in their patients' interests." "The physician's primary duty is to serve people."

Surgeons in an attempt to reduce pain and trauma, now endeavor to perform operations as fast and as accurately as possible. They have further modified the techniques of operations to accommodate the special characteristics of acupuncture anesthesia. Only through the combined efforts of all health personnel and full understanding on the part of the patient can acupuncture anesthesia be successful.

CHAPTER XV

ASSESSMENT OF ACUPUNCTURE ANESTHESIA

Since 1958 more than 400,000 operations have been performed in China using acupuncture anesthesia. The method is reported in use in 9 out of 10 hospitals with surgical departments in Shanghai. The successful operations carried out under acupuncture anesthesia include craniotomies with removal of large brain tumors, pneumonectomies, mitral commissurotomies, esophagogastrectomies for esophageal carcinoma, and all types of abdominal surgery. Acupuncture anesthesia has been used on patients of all ages from a two-day-old baby to an 90-year-old man. It has also been used in patients in shock or in deep coma. The rate of success has been reported to be as high as 90 percent. It is indeed a breakthrough in surgical anesthesia.

There are many advantages to acupuncture anesthesia. First, it is simple and economical. It does not require any complicated machines or apparatus. The needles and the electric stimulating machine may be possessed by a simple clinic or paramedical personnel. Because it introduces no medicine, it is inexpensive. The method is, therefore, particularly useful in distant and rural areas and under war conditions.

Secondly, since the patient is fully conscious during operations, many examinations can be carried out which might not be possible under conventional anesthesia. For example, in operations to correct squinting, when conventional anesthesia is given, the success and failure of the operation is known only after the effects of the drugs have worn off. With acupuncture anesthesia, however, the patient's eyeballs function normally and the surgeon may be able to evaluate his result immediately. A case in point is an operation on the thyroid. If the patient is able to talk during the operation, the surgeon would be able to compare the patient's speech and make sure that the recurrent laryngeal nerve was not damaged. In cases of plastic operations involving repair of tendons and muscles, it would indeed be a great advantage if the patient were able to be mobile at all times. The surgeon could not only find the injured tendons and muscles much more easily but also test the results of the operation immediately.

Thirdly, acupuncture anesthesia permits the normal physiological functioning of the patient to continue. The vital signs, including blood pressure, pulse, and respiration remain normal during the operation. After the operation, the healing of incisions and restoration of various functions of the internal organs are usually fast and satisfactory. Evidence further suggests that the function of normal immune mechanisms is not reduced and phagocytosis by leukocytes is not inhibited during acupuncture anesthesia as they are during conventional anesthesia. For this reason, postoperative infection seldom occurs.

The greatest advantage of acupuncture anesthesia lies in the fact that it may be used in debilitated and weak patients who may not be able to tolerate general anesthesia.

Nevertheless, acupuncture anesthesia is not without its drawbacks. Often its analgesic effect is not complete, and the patient may still experience pain during the operation to a certain degree. In addition, during abdominal operations, some patients may feel the pulling and pushing of internal organs, a quite uncomfortable experience. During thyroidectomy, if the huge thyroid gland has already pressed on the trachea, there may be danger of tracheal or larynegeal obstruction. During tonsillectomy, excessive blood loss is an annoying occurrence. It not only obscures the operative field, but also causes repeated gag reflexes of the pharynx. The gag reflexes may be greatly reduced if the patient on the day before tonsillectomy, practices to use a tongue depressor on the posterior part of his tongue. Further research and refinement of acupuncture anesthesia are still necessary.

APPENDIX I

NAME AND LOCATION OF POINTS

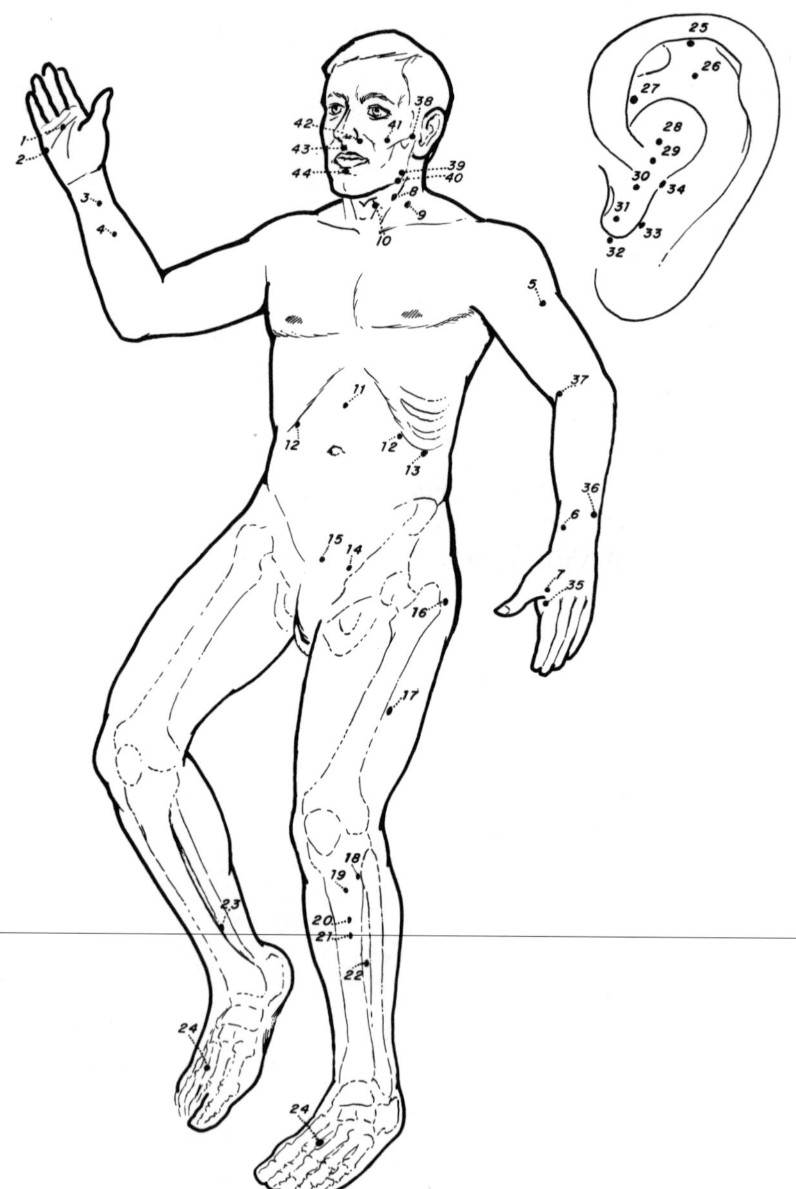

Fig. 11 Diagram showing 45 commonly-used points.

APPENDIX I

NAME AND LOCATION OF POINTS[74]

(Fig. 11)

No.	Name	Location
1.	Ya-tung	Between the third and fourth metacarpal, 1 inch from the digital fold
2.	Hou-hsi	Hold in half fist. Lateral aspect of the fifth metacarpal, on the horizontal fissure of palm
3.	Nei-kuan	Midline over the palmar aspect of forearm, 2 inches above the fold of the wrist, between two tendons
4.	Hung-men	Midline over the palmar aspect of forearm, 5 inches above the fold of the wrist, between two tendons
5.	Pi-ju	Outer aspect of upper arm, slightly anterior to the tip of deltoid muscle
6.	Lieh-chueh	Area of depression reached by the tip of the index finger of the physician during handshake. 1.5 inches above the radial prominence or the fold of wrist joint
7.	Ho-ku	In the skin web between the thumb and index finger. Midway between the junction of the first and second metacarpal and the fold, slightly toward the index finger
8.	Pien-tao	Below the angle of mandible, anterior to carotid artery

9.	Fu-tu	3 inches lateral to the thyroid cartilage. Between the sternal and clavicular insertions of the sternocleiodomastoid muscle
10.	Hung-yin	Half-inch lateral to thyroid cartilage
11.	Kuan-men	3 inches above and lateral to umbilicus
12.	Chang-men	Slightly below the tip of the 11th floating rib
13.	Tai-mo	Just below the costal margin of the 11th rib, on the same level as umbilicus
14.	Wei-tao	Below and anterior to the anterior superior iliac spine
15.	Tzu-kung	Midline of abdomen, 5 inches below umbilicus
16.	Huna-tiao	Posterior to the greater trochanter of femur. Depressed area in the gluteal fold when the individual is standing
17.	Feng-shih	Outer aspect of thigh on standing. The point reached by the top of middle finger of a loosely-hanging arm
18.	Chang-ling-chuan	Obtained when the knee is bent. Depressed area over the outer aspect of lower leg, below the anterior margin of head of fibula
19.	Tsu-san-li	3 inches below the patella of the knee joint. One finger-breadth lateral over the outer aspect of tibia
20.	Lan-wei	2 inches below point 19 on the outer aspect of tibia

21.	Shang-chu-hsu	3 inches below point 19 on the outer aspect of tibia
22.	Kuang-ming	5 inches above the lateral aspect of ankle joint
23.	San-yang-chiao	3 inches above the inner aspect of ankle joint, along the posterior edge of tibia
24.	Tai-chung	Dorsum of foot between the first and second toe, 1.5 inches behind the interdigital fold
25.	Lan-wei	Superior portion of helix
26.	Shen-men	Upper crus of anthelix, near the scaphoid fossa
27.	Chiao-kan	Triangular fossa
28.	Chang	Lower crus of anthelix
29.	Wei	Flat part of crus of helix
30.	Fei	Lower part of concha
31.	San-chiao	Lower part of concha
32.	Pi-chih-hsia	Incisura intertragica
33.	Nao-kan	In the groove between anthelix and helix
34.	Ya-tung	Inner aspect of point 33, in the groove between anthelix and helix
35.	San-chien	A depression at the radial aspect of the junction between the index finger and the second metacarpal
36.	Tzu-kou	Midline over the dorsal aspect of forearm, 3 inches above the folds of the wrist, between radius and ulna
37.	Chih-che	Slightly lateral to the center of cubital fold. Radial side of biceps tendon

38. Hsia-kuan	Depressed area behind the lower edge of the zygomatic arch and in front of the head of mandible. Obtained with mouth closed
39. Chia-tung	One finger-breadth anterior and superior to the angle of mandible. Muscular prominence during mastication
40. Ta-yin	Half-inch anterior to point 39. Depressed area along the posterior lower edge of mandible when the cheek is blown out with mouth closed
41. Chuan-liao	Below the outer canthus of eye. Depressed area over the lower edge of zygomatic arch
42. Yin-hsiang	2 inches below the inner canthus of eye, same level as tip of nose
43. Jen-chung	Junction between the upper and middle third of the nasolabial fold
44. Chen-chiang	Depressed area midway between the chin and lower lip
45. Feng-chih (Not shown in diagram)	Depressed area lateral to ligmentum flavum under the occipital bone in the posterior aspect of neck. On the same level as the lower margin of the mastoid prominence

APPENDIX II

ELECTRONIC STIMULATORS

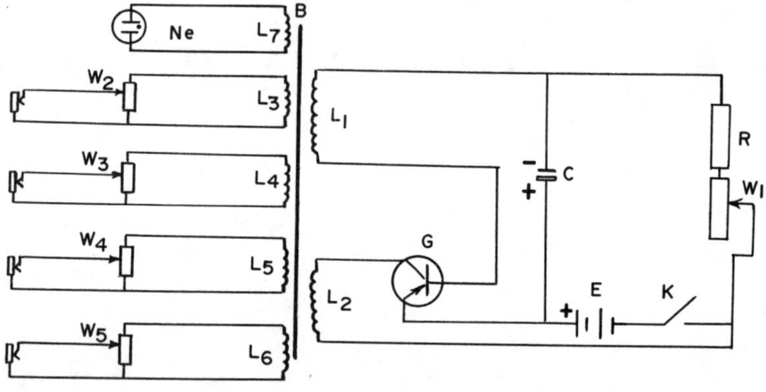

BT-701 STIMULATOR

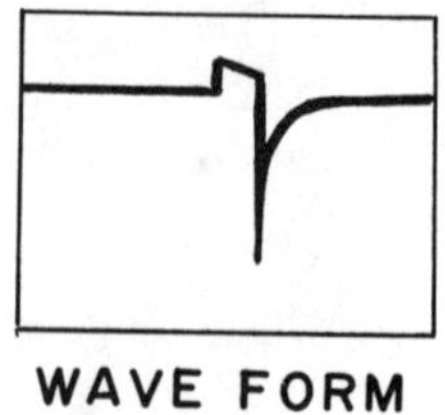

WAVE FORM

Fig. 12 Electronic Circuit and Wave Form of BT-701 Stimulator

APPENDIX II

ELECTRONIC STIMULATORS

The electronic circuitry of an acupuncture stimulator is not complicated. There are two models widely used in China. The effectiveness of these units has been attested by long successful experience in acupuncture anesthesia. Their circuits and specifications are briefly described as follows:

A. BT-701 Stimulator (Fig. 12)

1. Specifications:

The wave form is biphasic and pointed, as shown in the diagram. Pulse frequency varies from 120 to 2400 cycles per minute. Without load, output potential varies from 0 to 70 volts.

2. Parts:

E: 6 volt battery, consisting of four D-cells.
R: 2000 ohm resistor.
C: 10 volt, 20 uf electrolytic capacitor.
W_1: 47,000 ohm potentiometer with switch.
W_2, W_3, W_4 and W_5: 10,000 ohm potentiometer.
BG: 3AD6 power transistor.
B: Coil L_3:L_2:L_1 = 12:1:3. Coils L_3, L_4, L_5, L_6 and L_7 represent 1200 rounds of 0.07 millimeter of lacquer wire (LW); Coil L_1, 300 rounds of 0.10 millimeter of LW; Coil L_2, 100 rounds of 0.35 millimeter LW. The core consists of 0.35 millimeter thick D42 E-shaped silicon steel plates.
Ne: Neon bulb.

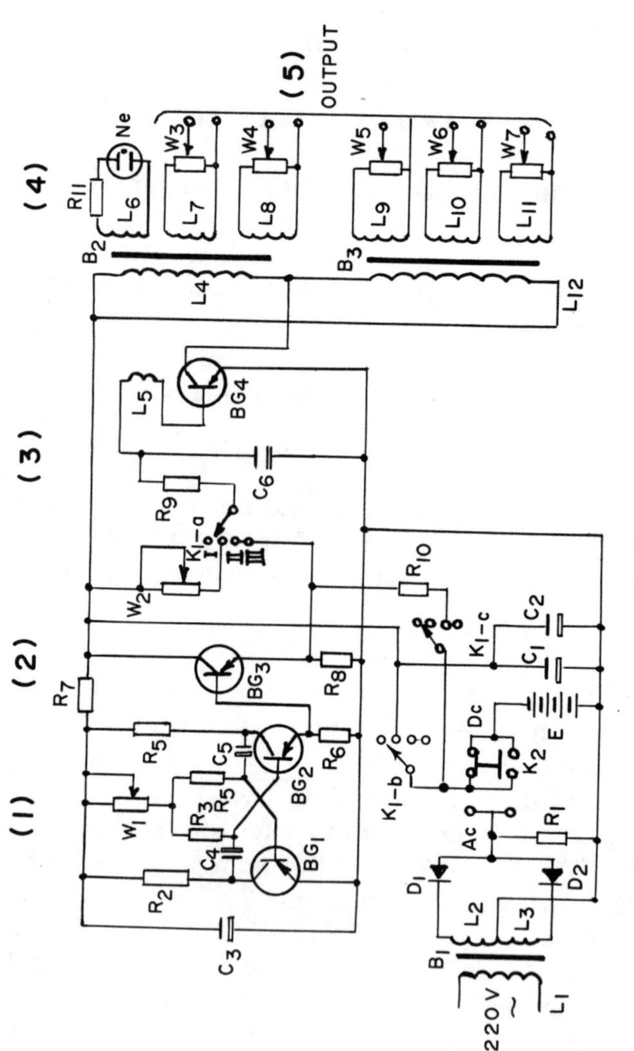

Fig. 13 Electronic Circuit of G6805 Stimulator

B. G6805 Stimulator (Fig. 13)

1. Specifications:

Continuous wave:

Frequency: 160 to 5000 cycles per minute.
Intensity: Positive pulse: 50 volts.
Negative pulse: 35 volts
Pulse width: Positive pulse: 0.5 msec.
Negative pulse: 0.25 msec.

Variable interval wave:

Frequency: 14 to 26 cycles per minute.
Intensity: Positive pulse: 50 volts.
Negative pulse: 35 volts.
Pulse width: Positive pulse: 0.5 msec.
Negative pulse: 0.25 msec.

Interrupted wave:

Frequency: 14 to 26 cycles per minute.
Intensity: Positive pulse: 50 volts.
Negative pulse: 35 volts.
Pulse width: Positive pulse: 0.5 msec.
Negative pulse: 0.25 msec.

2. Explanations: (Fig. 13)

(1) Multifrequency oscillator
(2) Output circuit
(3) Pulse oscillator
(4) Output monitor
(5) Output

3. Parts:

E: 6 volt battery, consisting of four D-cells.
R_1: 200 ohm 1/8 w resistor.
R_2, R_5: 2,000 ohm 1/8 w resistor.

R_3, R_4: 18,000 ohm 1/8 w resistor
R_6: 750 ohm 1/8 w resistor
R_7, R_9: 1000 ohm 1/8 w resistor
R_8: 2700 ohm 1/8 w resistor
R_{10}: 12,000 ohm 1/8 w resistor
R_{11}: 6,800 ohm 1/8 w resistor
W_1: 47,000 ohm potentiometer
W_2 to W_7: 22,000 ohm potentiometer
D_1, D_2: Diode 2 cp21A.
BG_1, BG_2, BG_3: Transistor 3AX31.
BG_4: Power transistor 3AD6.
C_1, C_2: 10 volt 200 uf electrolytic capacitor
C_3, C_4, C_5: 10 volt 100 uf electrolytic capacitor
C_6: ,10 volt 20 uf electrolytic capacitor
Ne: NHO-4C Neon bulb.
K_1: 3 x 4 band switch.
K_2: 2 x 2 tobbler switch.
B_2, B_3: Coil L_4 represents 55 rounds of 0.35 millimeter LW; L_5, 150 rounds of 0.10 millimeter LW; L_6, 3000 rounds of 0.05 millimeter LW; L_{12}, 55 rounds of 0.35 millimeter LW; L_7 to L_{11}, 1000 rounds of 0.1 millimeter LW. The core consists of 0.35 millimeter thick, D42 E-shaped silicon steel plates.
B_1: Coil L_1 represents 4830 rounds of 0.095 millimeter LW; L_2, L_3, 290 rounds of 0.35 millimeter LW. The core consists of 0.35 millimeter thick D42 E-shaped silicon steel plates.

REFERENCES

1. Veith, I.: *The Yellow Emperor's Classic of Internal Medicine.* University of California Press, Berkeley, 1972.
2. Palos, S.: *The Chinese Art of Healing.* Herder and Herder, New York, 1971.
3. Moss, L.: *Acupuncture and You.* Dell Publishing Co., New York, 1964.
4. Mann, F.: *The Ancient Art of Healing. Acupuncture.* Random House, Inc., 1963.
5. Austin, M.: *The Textbook of Acupuncture Therapy.* ASI Publishers, Inc., New York, 1972.
6. Wallnofer, H. and Rottauscher, A.: *Chinese Folk Medicine.* New American Library, Inc., New York, 1972.
7. *Some Basic Facts, Acupuncture Historic Background, Theory, Techniques, Actual Cases of Use It Works.* Maud Russell, Publisher, New York, 1972.
8. Turnberg, L.A.: Pins and Needles. *Manchester Med Gazette* 45: 16-20, 1966.
9. Huard, P. and Wong, M.: Present-day Trends in Acupuncture. *World Med J* 9: 335-336, 1962.
10. Ching, C.K.: The History and Romance of Acupuncture. *Med J Malaya* 18: 16-18, 1963.
11. Kee, C.P.: Acupuncture – An Ancient Chinese Art of Healing. *Singapore Med J* 4: 151-157, 1963.
12. Huard, P. and Wong, M.: *Chinese Medicine,* World University Library, McGraw-Hill Book Co., New York, 1968.
13. Grall, Y., Bornstein, S. and Fessard, J.: Acupuncture. From the Ancestral Treatment to Present Research. *Maroc (Casablanca)* 43: 979-982, 1964.
14. Matsumoto, T.: Acupuncture and US Medicine, *JAMA* 220: 1010, 1972.

15. Dimond, E.G.: Acupuncture Anesthesia. Western Medicine and Chinese Traditional Medicine, *JAMA* 218: 1558-1563, 1971.
16. Rich, N.M. and Dimond, F.C.: Results of Vietnamese Acupuncture Seen at the Second Surgical Hospital. *Milit Med* 132: 791-795, 1967.
17. Johnson, J.B.: Office Rounds with an Acupuncture in Saigon. *Med Ann D C* 34: 287-289, 1965.
18. Dimond, E.G.: Ward Round with an Acupuncturist. *New Eng J Med* 272: 575-577 (Mar. 18,) 1965.
19. Elliott, F.A.: Acupuncture and Other Forms of Counter-irritation. *Trans College of Physicians of Philadelphia* 30: 81-84, 1962.
20. Altekruse, E.B.: The Emergence and Re-emergence of Acupuncture – A Chinese Medical Method. *Stanford Med Bulletin* 20: 117-124, 1962.
21. Veith, I.: Acupuncture Therapy – Past and Present. *JAMA* 180: 478-484 (May 12) 1962.
22. *Acupuncture and Moxubustion.* The Academy Press Co., Kowloon, Hong Kong, 1971.
23. *Acupuncture and Moxubustion.* People's Publishing Co., Peking, China, 1970.
24. Shanghai Medical College No. 1: *Fundamental Knowledge of Chinese Medicine, Modern Therapy and Herb Medicine.* People's Publishing Co., Shanghai, China, 1971.
25. Shanghai Medical College No. 2: *Handbook of Internal Medicine.* People's Publishing Co., Shanghai, China, 1971.
26. Perkins, J.J.: *Principles and Methods of Sterilization in Health Sciences.* C.C Thomas, Springfield, Illinois, 1969.
27. Alexander, E.L., Burley, W., Ellison D., and Valleri, R.: *Care of the Patient in Surgery, including Techniques.* CV Mosby Co., St. Louis, 1967.
28. Figar, S., Drejci, D. and Tuhacek, M.: Vasomotor Reactions Following Acupuncture in Lumbosacral Syndromes. *Cesk Oftalmol* 27: 251-255, 1964.

29. LaBrooy, E.B.: Counter-Irritation Marks Produced by Traditional Chinese Medical Practice. Their Recognition and Distinction from Homicidal Injuries. *J Forensic Med* 10: 94-103, 1965.
30. Fukuda, K., Kiriyama, T., Kashiwagi, T., Okita, J., Doganemaru, T. and Sakotoku, J.: Foreign Bodies (Acupuncture Needles) in the Kidney Combined with a Stone: Report of a Case. *Acta Urol Jap (Kyoto)* 15: 223-236, 1969.
31. Asano, K.: Foreign Body Granuloma Caused by a Broken Silver Needle for Acupuncture. *Otolaryngology (Tokyo)* 41: 289-291, 1969.
32. Schiff, A.F.: A Fatality Due to Acupuncture. *Med Times* 93: 630-631, 1965.
33. *Acupuncture Anesthesia.* Foreign Languages Press. Peking, 1972.
34. Shanghai Cooperative Group of Acupuncture Anesthesia: Why Operation Can be Performed Under Acupuncture Anesthesia? *Red Flag Magazine* No. 9, 1971.
35. People's Liberation Army General Hospital: A Few Concepts about the Principles of Acupuncture Anesthesia. *Red Flag Magazine* No. 9, 1971.
36. Shanghai Psychiatric Hospital: Treatment of Psychiatric Diseases with Acupuncture. A Method Inspired by Acupuncture Anesthesia. *Liberation Daily News,* Jan. 22, 1972.
37. People's Liberation Army General Hospital, Canton Division: Discussion of Principles of Pain Relief with Acupuncture Anesthesia. *Red Flag Magazine* No. 9, 1971.
38. Shanghai Medical College No. 1. Affiliating Chung-San Memorial Hospital: Acupuncture Anesthesia Group. Study of Relations between the Acupuncture Points and Surrounding Nervous Structure by Anatomical Dissection. *Liberation Daily News,* January 5, 1972.

39. Chinese Liberation Army, 245 Division, Acupuncture Anesthesia Group No. 1: Do Not Overlook the Function of Sympathetic Nervous System in Pain Relief with Acupuncture Anesthesia. *Liberation Daily News,* January 5, 1972.
40. Shanghai Medical College No. 1 Acupuncture Anesthesia Group: Discussion of Principles of Facial and Nasal Needles for Acupuncture Anesthesia. *Liberation Daily News* Jan. 5, 1972.
41. Chiang, S.Y.: My Understanding of Ear Needles for Acupuncture Anesthesia. *Liberation Daily News,* January 5, 1972.
42. International Peace Hospital for Women and Children. Acupuncture Anesthesia Group: The Relation Between Ear Needles and Nervous System. *Liberation Daily News,* March 19, 1972.
43. Hsing, C.: Specificity and Nonspecificity of Acupuncture Points. *Liberation Daily News* December 23, 1971.
44. Kuang-Si Medical College Acupuncture Anesthesia Research Group: Activities of the Reticular Formation of The Brain Stem Under Acupuncture Anesthesia. *Kuang-Ming Daily News* January 31, 1972.
45. Wolff, H.G. and Wolff, S.: *Pain.* C. C Thomas, Springfield, Illinois, 1948 and 1958.
46. Crosby, E.C., Humphrey, T. and Lauer, E.W.: *Correlative Anatomy of the Nervous System.* The Macmillan Company, New York, 1962.
47. Crue, B.L.: *Pain and Suffering. Selected Aspects.* C. C Thomas, Springfield, Illinois, 1970.
48. Chang, H.T.: The Struggle between Painful and Nonpainful Sensation in Acupuncture Anesthesia. *Liberation Daily News,* December 2, 1971.
49. Sinclair, D.C.: Cutaneous Sensation and the Doctrine of Specific Energy. *Brain* 78: 584-614, 1955.

50. Jones, M.H.: Second Pain: Fact or Artefact? *Science* 124: 442-443, 1956.
51. Grinker, R.R. and Sahs, A.L.: *Neurology. C. C Thomas* Springfield, Illinois, 1966.
52. Melzack, R. and Wall, P.D.: Pain Mechanisms: A New Theory. *Science* 150: 971-979, 1965.
53. Henry Ford Hospital International Symposium: *Pain.* Edited by Knighton, R.S. and Dumke, P.R. J. & A. Churchill Ltd. London, 1966.
54. Personal communication. Edinger, H.M.
55. Wall, P.D. and Sweet, W.H.: Temporary Abolition of Pain in Man. *Science* 155: 108-109, 1967.
56. Sweet, W.H., and Wepsic, J.G.: Treatment of Chronic Pain by Stimulation of Fibers of Primary Afferent Neuron. *Trans Amer Neurol Assoc* 93: 103-107, 1968.
57. White, J.C. and Sweet, W.H.: *Pain and the Neurosurgeons. A Forty-Year Experience.* C. C Thomas, Springfield, Illinois, 1969. Chapter XIX Control of Pain by Activation of Inhibitory Mechanisms, p. 888-904.
58. Shealy, C.N.: Dorsal Column Electrohypalgesia. *Headache.* 9: 99-102, 1969.
59. Shealy, C.N., Mortimer, J.T. and Hagfors, N.R.: Dorsal Column Electroanalgesia *J Neurosurg* 32, 560-564, 1970.
60. Hosobuchi, Y., Adams, J.E., and Weinstein, P.R.,: Preliminary Percutaneous Dorsal Column Stimulation Prior to Permanent Implantation. *J Neurosurg* 37: 242, 1972.
61. Notermans, S.L.H.: Measurement of the Pain Threshold, Determined by Electrical Stimulation and its Clinical Application. Part I: Methods and Factors Possibly Influencing the Pain Threshold. *Neurology* 16: 1071-1086, 1966.
62. Notermans, S.L.H.: Measurement of the Pain Threshold, Determined by Electrical Stimulation and its Clinical Application. Part II: Clinical Application in Neurological and Neurosurgical Patients. *Neurology* 17: 58-73, 1967.

63. Breenan, R.W., Nelson, P.B., et. al., Somatic Sensory Changes During Dorsal Column Stimulation. *Neurology* 22: 437, 1972.
64. Nashold, B.S. and Friedman, H.: Dorsal Column Stimulation for Control of Pain. *J Neurosurg* 36: 590, 1972.
65. Meyer, G.A., and Fields, H.L.: Causalgia Treated by Selective Large Fiber Stimulation of Peripheral Nerve. *Brain* 95: 163, 1972.
66. Sheldon, C.H., Pudenz, R.H. and Bullara, L.: Development and Clinical Capabilities of a New Implantable Biostimulator. *Amer J Surgery* 124: 212-217, 1972.
67. Valery, L.P.: Homeopathy and Acupuncture. The Possibilities of Homeopathy in Cardiac Diseases. Preparation of the Patient for Odono-Stomatologic Interventions. *Chir Dentist France* 38: 25-26, 1968.
68. Schwartz, E.: Dentistry and Electroacupuncture, *Zahnaerzti Mitt (Koln)* 57: 17-18, 1967.
69. Valery, L.P.: Additional Information on the Practice of Acupuncture. Localization of Points, the Punctometer-Galvano Puncture. *Chir Dentist France* 36: 37-41, 1966.
70. Pavlik, L., Umlauf, R., Rafaj, J. and Odehnal, F.: Our Experience with Acupuncture in Otorhinolaryngology. Preliminary Report. *Cesk Otolaryngol (Praha)* 15: 164-168, 1966.
71. Bischdo, J.: The Possibility of Acupuncture in the Ear, Nose and Throat Area. *Monatsschr Ohrenheilkd Laryngorhinol* 97: 465-467, 1963.
72. Gorlina, A.A. Et. al: Use of Acupuncture for Post-Tonsillectomy Analgesia. *Vestn Otorinolaringol (Moskva)* 25: 48-50, 1963.
73. Chang, H.K.: Chest Pain after Pneumonectomy Treated by Acupuncture. *Zhonghua Waike Zazki (Peking)* 9: 389-390, 1961.
74. *Diagram of Acupuncture Points.* People's Health Publishing Co., Canton, China, 1971.

INDEX

AVAILABLE AT YOUR LOCAL BOOKSTORE
OR USE THIS ORDER FORM

MEDICAL EXAMINATION PUBLISHING CO., INC.
65-36 Fresh Meadow Lane, Flushing, N.Y. 11365

Date: ____________

Please send me the following books:

____

____

____

____

____

☐ Payment enclosed to save postage.

☐ Bill me. I will remit payment within 30 days.

Name ______________________________________

Address ____________________________________

City & State ________________________ Zip ________
(Please print)

OTHER BOOKS AVAILABLE

ITEMS	Code	Unit Price
MEDICAL EXAM REVIEW BOOKS		
Vol. 1 Comprehensive	101	$12.00
Vol. 2 Clinical Medicine	102	7.50
Vol. 2A Txtbk. Study Guide of Int. Med.	123	7.50
Vol. 2B Txtbk. Study Guide of Int. Med.	130	7.50
Vol. 3 Basic Sciences	103	7.50
Vol. 4 Obstetrics-Gynecology	104	7.50
Vol. 4A Textbk. Study Guide of Gynecology	152	7.50
Vol. 5 Surgery	105	7.50
Vol. 5A Textbk. Study Guide of Surgery	150	7.50
Vol. 6 Public Health & Prev. Medicine	106	7.50
Vol. 8 Psychiatry & Neurology	108	7.50
Vol.11 Pediatrics	111	7.50
Vol.12 Anesthesiology	112	7.50
Vol.13 Orthopaedics	113	10.00
Vol.14 Urology	114	10.00
Vol.15 Ophthalmology	115	10.00
Vol.16 Otolaryngology	116	10.00
Vol.17 Radiology	117	10.00
Vol.18 Thoracic Surgery	118	10.00
Vol.19 Neurological Surgery	119	15.00
Vol.20 Physical Medicine	128	10.00
Vol.21 Dermatology	127	10.00
Vol.22 Gastroenterology	141	10.00
Vol.23 Child Psychiatry	126	10.00
Vol.24 Pulmonary Diseases	143	10.00
Vol.25 Nuclear Medicine	133	10.00
Vol.26 Allergy	132	10.00
Vol.27 Plastic Surgery	129	10.00
Vol.28 Cardiovascular Diseases	138	10.00
Vol.29 Oncology	146	10.00
ECFMG Exam Review - Part One	120	7.50
ECFMG Exam Review - Part Two	121	7.50
BASIC SCIENCE REVIEW BOOKS		
Anatomy Review	201	7.00
Biochemistry Review	202	7.00
Digestive System Basic Sciences	215	7.00
Heart & Vascular Systems Basic Sciences	212	7.00
Microbiology Review	203	7.00
Nervous System Basic Sciences	210	7.00
Pathology Review	204	7.00
Pharmacology Review	205	7.00
Physiology Review	206	7.00
Respiratory System Basic Sciences	213	7.00
Urinary System B.Sci.	214	7.00
Anatomy Textbook Study Guide	124	7.00
Histology Textbook Study Guide	151	7.00
Medical Physiology Textbk. Study Guide	155	7.00
SPECIALTY BOARD REVIEW BOOKS		
Dermatology Specialty Board Review	311	10.00
Family Practice Specialty Board Review	309	10.00
Internal Medicine Specialty Board Review	303	10.00
Neurology Specialty Board Review	306	10.00
Obstetrics-Gynecology Spec. Bd. Review	304	10.00
Pathology Specialty Board Review	305	10.00
Pediatrics Specialty Board Review	301	10.00
Psychiatry Specialty Board Review	312	10.00
Surgery Specialty Board Review	302	10.00
The Otolaryngology Boards	313	10.00
The Psychiatry Boards	307	8.00

ITEMS	Code	Unit Price
STATE BOARD REVIEW BOOKS		
Med. State Brd. Rev. - Basic Sciences	411	$9.00
Med. State Brd. Rev. - Clinical Sciences	412	9.00
Cardiopulmonary Techn. Exam. Rev. - Vol. 1	473	7.50
Cytology Exam. Review Book - Vol. 1	454	7.50
Dental Exam. Review Book - Vol. 1	431	7.50
Dental Exam. Review Book - Vol. 2	432	7.50
Dental Exam. Review Book - Vol. 3	433	7.50
Dental Hygiene Exam. Review - Vol. 1	461	7.50
Emergency Med. Techn. Exam. Rev. - Vol. 1	465	7.50
Emergency Med. Techn. Exam. Rev. - Vol. 2	466	7.50
Immunology Exam. Review Book - Vol. 1	424	7.50
Inhalation Therapy Exam. Review - Vol. 1	471	7.50
Inhalation Therapy Exam. Review - Vol. 2	344	7.50
Laboratory Asst. Exam. Rev. Bk. - Vol. 1	455	7.50
Medical Librarian Exam. Rev. Bk. - Vol. 1	495	7.50
Medical Record Library Science - Vol. 1	496	7.50
Medical Techn. Exam. Review - Vol. 1	451	7.50
Medical Techn. Exam. Review - Vol. 2	452	7.50
Occupational Therapy Exam. Rev. - Vol. 1	475	7.50
Optometry Exam. Review	469	10.00
Pharmacy Exam. Review Book - Vol. 1	421	7.50
Physical Therapy Exam. Review - Vol. 1	481	7.50
Physical Therapy Exam. Review - Vol. 2	482	7.50
X-Ray Technology Exam. Rev. - Vol. 1	441	7.50
X-Ray Technology Exam. Rev. - Vol. 2	442	7.50
X-Ray Technology Exam. Rev. - Vol. 3	443	7.50
NURSING EXAM REVIEW BOOKS		
Vol. 1 Medical-Surgical Nursing	501	4.50
Vol. 2 Psychiatric-Mental Health Nursing	502	4.50
Vol. 3 Maternal-Child Health Nursing	503	4.50
Vol. 4 Basic Sciences	504	4.50
Vol. 5 Anatomy and Physiology	505	4.50
Vol. 6 Pharmacology	506	4.50
Vol. 7 Microbiology	507	4.50
Vol. 8 Nutrition & Diet Therapy	508	4.50
Vol. 9 Community Health	509	4.50
Vol.10 History & Law of Nursing	510	4.50
Vol.11 Fundamentals of Nursing	511	4.50
Practical Nursing Examination Rev. - Vol. 1	711	4.50
CASE STUDY BOOKS		
Allergy Case Studies	027	10.00
Cardiology Case Studies	001	10.00
Chest Diseases Case Studies	012	10.00
Child Psychiatry Case Studies	029	10.00
Cutaneous Medicine Case Studies	014	7.50
ECG Case Studies	003	7.50
Endocrinology Case Studies	008	10.00
Gastroenterology Case Studies	004	10.00
Hematology Case Studies	020	10.00
Infectious Diseases Case Studies	011	7.50
Neurology Case Studies	006	10.00
Orthopedic Surgery Case Studies	030	10.00
Otolaryngology Case Studies	021	10.00
Pediatric Hematology Case Studies	018	10.00
Pediatric Oculo-Neural Dis. Case Studies	023	10.00
Respiratory Care Case Studies	019	7.50
Urology Case Studies	017	10.00
MEDICAL OUTLINE SERIES		
Cancer Chemotherapy	631	10.00
Child Psychiatry	613	10.00

Prices subject to change.

OTHER BOOKS AVAILABLE

ITEMS	Code	Unit Price
MEDICAL OUTLINE SERIES *(Cont'd.)*		
Endocrinology	614	$10.00
Histology	662	8.00
Otolaryngology	661	8.00
Psychiatry	621	8.00
Urology	611	8.00
SELF-ASSESSMENT BOOKS		
Self-Assess. Cur. Knldge - Biochemistry	266	7.50
S.A.C.K. in Cardiovascular Diseases	275	10.00
S.A.C.K. in Diagnostic Radiology	278	10.00
S.A.C.K. in Family Practice	261	10.00
S.A.C.K. in Infectious Diseases	263	10.00
S.A.C.K. in Internal Medicine	257	10.00
S.A.C.K. in Neurology	254	10.00
S.A.C.K. for Nurse Anesthetist	715	7.50
S.A.C.K. in Obstet./Gynecology	260	10.00
S.A.C.K. in O.R. Techn.	474	7.50
S.A.C.K. in Otolaryngology	270	10.00
S.A.C.K. in Pathology	253	10.00
S.A.C.K. in Pediatrics	256	10.00
S.A.C.K. in Psychiatry	252	10.00
S.A.C.K. in Pulmonary Diseases	271	10.00
S.A.C.K. in Rheumatology	258	10.00
S.A.C.K. in Surgery	250	10.00
S.A.C.K. in Surgery for Family Physicians	259	10.00
S.A.C.K. in Urology	251	10.00
S.A.C.K. in X-Ray Tech.	274	7.50
MEDICAL HANDBOOKS		
E.N.T. Emergencies	639	8.00
Medical Emergencies	635	8.00
Neurology	604	8.00
Obstetrical Emergencies	634	8.00
Ophthalmologic Emergencies	633	8.00
Pediatric Anesthesia	637	8.00
Pediatric Neurology	636	10.00
PRACTICAL POINTS BOOKS		
In Anesthesiology	700	10.00
In Gastroenterology	733	7.00
In Pediatrics	702	10.00
PRACTITIONERS GUIDES		
OB-Gynecology Disorders	704	10.00
Ophthalmologic Disorders	703	10.00
JOURNAL ARTICLE COMPILATIONS		
Ambulance Service Journal Articles	517	10.00
Blood Banking & Immunohemat. Jour. Art.	798	10.00
Emergency Room Journal Articles	795	8.00
Hodgkin's Disease Journal Articles	515	12.00
Hosp. & Inst. Eng. & Maintenance J. Art.	793	8.00
Hosp. Electronic Data Process. J. Art.	791	8.00
Hosp. Pharmacy Journal Articles	799	10.00
Hosp. Security & Safety Journal Articles	796	8.00
Human Cytomegalovirus Journal Articles	522	15.00
Immunosuppressive Therapy Journal Art.	526	20.00

ITEMS	Code	Unit Price
Institutional Laundry Journal Articles	789	$18.00
Lithium & Psychiatry Journal Articles	520	15.00
Psychosomatic Medicine Current J. Art.	788	12.00
Outpatient Services Journal Articles, 2nd Ed.	797	10.00
Outpatient Services Journal Articles, *1st Ed.*	794	8.00
Selected Papers in Inhalation Therapy	523	10.00
TYPIST HANDBOOKS		
Medical Typist's Guide for Hx & Phys.	976	4.50
Radiology Typist Handbook	981	4.50
Surgical Typist Handbook	991	4.50
Transcribers Guide to Med. Terminology	973	4.50
ESSAY Q. & A. REVIEW BOOKS		
Blood Banking Principles Rev.	339	8.00
Cardiology Review	337	10.00
Colon & Rectal Surg. Cont. Ed. Rev.	338	10.00
Neurology Review	345	10.00
Obstet. Nursing Cont. Ed. Rev.	350	5.00
Ophthalmology Review	347	10.00
Orthopedics Review	349	10.00
Psychiatry Cont. Ed. Rev.	352	10.00
Psych./Mental Hlth. Nursing Cont. Ed. Rev.	351	5.00
OTHER BOOKS		
Acid Base Homeostasis	601	4.00
Allergy Annual Review	325	12.00
Bailey & Love's Short Practice of Surgery	900	20.00
Benign & Malignant Bladder Tumors	932	15.00
Blood Groups	860	2.50
Clinical Diagnostic Pearls	730	4.50
Concentrations of Solutions	602	3.00
Critical Care Manual	983	10.00
Cryogenics in Surgery	754	24.00
Diagnosis & Treatment of Breast Lesions	748	15.00
Emergency Care Manual	984	7.50
English-Spanish Guide for Med. Personnel	721	2.50
Fundamental Orthopedics	603	4.50
Guide to Medical Reports	962	4.50
Human Anatomical Terminology	982	3.00
Illustrated Laboratory Techniques	919	10.00
Introduction to Acupuncture	753	5.00
Introduction to Blood Banking	975	8.00
Introduction to the Clinical History	729	3.00
Lab. Diagnosis of Inf. Dis.	965	7.50
Math for Med Techs	964	7.00
Multilingual Guide for Medical Personnel	961	2.50
Neoplasms of the Gastrointestinal Tract	736	20.00
Neurophysiology Study Guide	600	7.00
Nursing & the Nephrology Patient	376	5.00
Outpatient Hemorrhoidectomy Lig. Tech.	752	12.50
Profiles in Surgery, Gynec. & Obstetrics	963	5.00
Radiological Physics Exam. Review	486	10.00
Skin, Heredity & Malignant Neoplasms	744	20.00
Testicular Tumors	743	20.00
Tissue Adhesives in Surgery	756	24.00
Understanding Hematology	977	8.00

Prices subject to change.